CHRISSY HARADA

Restoring Health & Vitality in Motherhood

A Holistic Guide to Healing Hormones, Energy & Wellbeing Naturally from the 4th Trimester & Beyond.

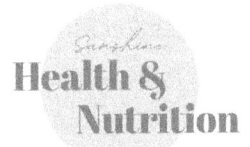

First published by Sunshine Health & Nutrition 2025

Copyright © 2025 by Chrissy Harada

All rights reserved. No part of this publication may be reproduced, stored or transmitted in any form or by any means, electronic, mechanical, photocopying, recording, scanning, or otherwise without written permission from the publisher. It is illegal to copy this book, post it to a website, or distribute it by any other means without permission.

Chrissy Harada has no responsibility for the persistence or accuracy of URLs for external or third-party Internet Websites referred to in this publication and does not guarantee that any content on such Websites is, or will remain, accurate or appropriate.

Medical Disclaimer

The information provided is for educational and informational purposes only and is not intended as medical advice. This information should not be used for diagnosing or treating any health condition or disease. Always consult a qualified healthcare professional for advice regarding any medical condition or treatment. Reliance on any information provided is solely at your own risk.

First edition

ISBN: 978-1-7637133-3-8

This book was professionally typeset on Reedsy. Find out more at reedsy.com

For every mother longing for more energy, vitality and well-being amidst the relentless demands of life – may the insights in these pages help you reclaim your health, extend your years and enrich the life you live.

Feeling well makes everyday life easier - more patience, more energy and more presence. Prioritizing your health and well-being is one of the most valuable gifts you can give to not only yourself but also your children.

— Chrissy Harada

Contents

Preface	v
A Note to You	v
Introduction	1
What You'll Get from This Book	1
The Myths Keeping You Stuck	2
Understanding Holistic Health: It's All Connected	3
The Transformative Experience of Motherhood	4
I Part One	
1 What is Postnatal Depletion?	9
Isn't this Just the Baby Blues?	10
The Truth is Recovery Takes Longer than We've Been Told	10
Recognizing the Signs of Postnatal Depletion	11
Understanding the Causes of Postnatal Depletion	16
Why Modern-Day Mothers Are More at Risk	20
Why Addressing Postnatal Depletion is Important	23
Postnatal Depletion vs. Postnatal Depression: Key Differences	24
Recovering from Postnatal Depletion	26
2 The Postpartum Hormonal Roller-Coaster	27
Signs Your Hormones Need Support After the 4th Trimester	28
Hormone Fluctuations and Underlying Health Conditions in Postpartum	33
Natural Ways to Restore Hormonal Balance	34
3 Nutritional Replenishment and the Impact of Vitamin and...	42

Why Nutrient Deficiencies Are the New Normal	43
Nutrients to Support Postnatal Depletion	45
What About Supplements?	49
The Broader Health Impacts of Nutritional Deficiencies	51
4 Restoring Gut Health	54
How Routine Antibiotics During Birth Can Disrupt the Gut	55
Common Signs of Poor Gut Health	56
Phase 1: Gentle Gut Restoration	57
Phase 2: Deeper Microbiome Restoration	60
5 Eating to Fight Chronic Inflammation	61
Why an Anti-Inflammatory Diet Matters After Birth	61
How an Anti-Inflammatory Diet Supports Postpartum Recovery	63
Inflammatory Foods to Avoid	63
6 Postnatal Meal Plan - 2 Weeks	68
Week 1	69
Week 2	71
Meal Plan Tips	73
7 The Mental and Emotional Load of Motherhood	75
Strategies & Tips	77
8 Navigating New Anxieties in Motherhood	79
How Nutrition Can Support Anxiety Management	80
9 Strategies for Sleep Struggles	86
Hormonal Changes	88
Lifestyle Factors	88
How to Improve Your Sleep	89
Natural Herbs and Supplements to Support Sleep (with Breastfeeding Considerations)	91
10 The Role of Exercise in Postpartum Recovery	94
Getting Started: Gentle Exercise for Postnatal Recovery	96

II Part Two

11 Balancing Hormones After the First Year	101
Why Are Hormones Still Out of Balance After the First Year of Motherhood?	102
Nourishing Your Hormones	105
Vitamins & Minerals that Nourish Hormones	108
Hormone Restoration Meal Plan	109
12 Stress Less by Controlling Cortisol	114
Could Your Cortisol Be Too High?	114
Why High Cortisol Is Harmful	115
Natural Ways to Reduce Cortisol	116
13 When PMS Returns — Causes & Holistic Relief	119
What Makes PMS Worse After Having a Baby?	120
Functional Medicine Approach to Postpartum PMS	121
Natural Remedies for PMS Relief	122
14 Health & Healing Begins in the Gut	125
Gut Health & Metabolism: More Than Just a Weight Issue	126
The Gut-Brain Connection: A New Lens on Mental Health	126
Immunity Starts in the Gut	127
Gut Health & Hormonal Balance: The Hidden Link	127
Gut Health & Aging: What Changes and Why It Matters	128
The Consequences of Poor Gut Health	129
15 Gut Health Restoration - Remove, Replace, Repair, Restore...	132
Step 1: Remove - Eliminating Gut Irritants	133
Step 2: Replace – Restore Digestive Support	138
Step 3: Repair – Healing the Gut Lining	139
Key Tools for Gut Lining Repair	140
Step 4: Restore — Rebuilding the Microbiome	143
16 Enhancing Your Energy	148
Natural Energy Boosters	149
17 Building a Robust Immune System	154
How a Healthy Gut Strengthens Your Immune System	155

Immune-Boosting Foods and Functional Ingredients	156
Immune-Boosting Meal Plan	159
18 What's on Your Plate? Why Organic Matters	164
How to Incorporate More Organic Foods Affordably	165
19 Reducing Harmful Chemicals - Safer Personal Care, Cleaning...	169
The Top Toxins to Eliminate	170
How to Reduce Chemicals in Your Diet	172
Reducing Chemical Exposure in Personal Care & Cleaning Products	175
Start Small - Choose One Area for Cleaner Swaps and Build	177
20 The Body's Detox Dilemma: Natural Systems vs. Synthetic...	179
Root Causes of Toxic Load and Detox Dysfunction	180
Methods of Detoxification	184
Parasites: The Hidden Saboteurs	188
Supporting the Liver	189
Bringing It All Together	192
21 Benefits of Personalized Nutrition & Health Plans	194
Test Don't Guess – Functional Tests	196
Gut Microbiome Testing	197
Hair Tissue Mineral Analysis (HTMA) Tests	198
22 Conclusion	201
Moving Forward with Confidence: Thriving in Motherhood	201
Scientific References	203
Thank You & A Small Request	262
About the Author	263
Also by Chrissy Harada	265

Preface

A Note to You

Welcome Mama,

I see you, I know how much you give, how much you care for your family and how little time you have to focus on yourself. If you're feeling depleted, struggling with brain fog, low energy, mood swings, poor sleep, anxiety, overwhelm, or a sense of losing a part of yourself since becoming a mother, you are not alone – and you are in the right place.

This book is here to guide you back to feeling like you again, and my hope is, that you feel better than ever. Using evidence-based strategies backed by over 440 scientific studies (references at the back), we'll explore practical, natural ways to restore your energy, balance your hormones, and support your mood and overall well-being. By the time you reach the last page, you'll have the knowledge and tools to rebuild your vitality and step into a healthier, more vibrant version of yourself – one that allows you to truly thrive in early motherhood and beyond.

Now, let's be real. Motherhood is incredible, but it can also be really hard to do properly. What no one told me when I first began this journey is just how much it would demand from me – physically, emotionally and mentally. And yet, far too many women suffer in silence, afraid to voice their struggles for fear of seeming ungrateful or like they're failing - almost as if it's secret woman's business. The reality is, much of your exhaustion, brain fog and overwhelm aren't just part of motherhood – they can also be signs of deep nutritional depletion, your body's way of calling for replenishment and self-care.

In my case, I was utterly depleted of nutrients because even though I had a great diet, I wasn't absorbing the nutrients properly due to poor gut health and my minerals levels were deranged. This affected my ability to handle stress, regulate my hormones and prevented my mind and body from functioning optimally. In effect making my introduction to becoming a mother much harder than it needed to be.

Research shows that **up to 50%–75% of new mothers experience some degree of postpartum distress and one in five develop postpartum depression or anxiety**. And that's only counting the women who seek help, I certainly didn't report my experience. Despite these numbers, societal pressure often makes us feel like we *should* be thriving. It is as if we are supposed to master motherhood overnight, whilst also dealing with sleep deprivation, depletion, wild hormone fluctuations, new routines and the identity shift that comes with motherhood. If you've gotten through the 4th trimester with your baby and are still feeling depleted, you might have postnatal depletion.

Postnatal depletion is a state of ongoing physical, emotional and mental exhaustion that can affect mothers for years after childbirth, often due to nutrient loss, hormonal shifts, sleep disruption, and the demands of caring for a baby. From a holistic perspective, it reflects the body's response to being under-supported and undernourished, requiring a whole-person approach to restore vitality.

No two motherhood journeys are the same, but one truth remains: every mother deserves to feel supported, nourished, and whole — in body, mind, and spirit. Your experience may look different from others', but your well-being is no less worthy of care. When you prioritize your health, you strengthen the foundation that lets you show up for your family with energy, joy and resilience.

Introduction

What You'll Get from This Book

As mothers, our health often determines the health and stability of the entire household. Prioritizing your own well-being isn't selfish, it's foundational. When you support yourself, you're not just improving your own quality of life, you're modeling resilience, self-respect, and vitality for your children. And when you feel well, you have more energy, patience, and clarity which creates a ripple effect and sets the tone for your family.

This book is your practical guide to understanding the root causes of postnatal depletion, hormonal imbalance, and persistent fatigue. Whether you're a few months postpartum or several years into motherhood, these challenges can linger quietly and go unaddressed for far too long. You may look fine on paper, but still feel off, rundown, or disconnected from the person you used to be.

With the right nutritional and holistic strategies, lifestyle support, and clarity about what's going on beneath the surface, healing is possible. You'll learn how to:

- Boost your energy and break free from chronic fatigue
- Nourish your body with the nutrients it actually needs
- Improve gut health and support natural detox pathways
- Simplify your approach to wellness so it fits into everyday life
- Sleep better and think more clearly, even in the chaos
- Lighten your mental load and reduce stress
- Create a low-tox home that supports your whole family's health

- Build lasting habits that strengthen your resilience over time

This isn't a quick fix or a one-size-fits-all protocol. It's a grounded, whole-body approach to healing, designed with real mothers and real lives in mind. If you've been told everything is "fine" when you know it's not, this book will help you connect the dots and take action with confidence.

It's the guide I wish I'd had in my own early years of motherhood, when I was exhausted, confused, and looking for answers. Whether you're in the thick of the fourth trimester or years down the track still wondering why you don't feel like yourself—this book is for you.

The Myths Keeping You Stuck

On your health journey, you've likely encountered these myths:

- That constant exhaustion is just an unavoidable part of growing older.
- That poor health is simply the hand you've been dealt – an outcome of bad luck or genetics.
- That feeling unwell is something you simply have to "push through"
- That your symptoms are unrelated to what you eat or how your gut functions
- That your diet has no real connection to your hormones.
- That your body should "just handle everything" on its own, without intentional care or support.

These beliefs aren't just outdated—they're unhelpful. They can keep you stuck, dismissing real symptoms and delaying the care you need. The truth is: your body may be giving you important signals and you don't have to ignore them.

Yes, motherhood demands a lot. But that doesn't mean struggling through it is a badge of honor. If you've ever tried to get help—talked to multiple doctors, described your fatigue, mood swings, or mental fog—only to hear,

INTRODUCTION

"Your labs are fine," or "It's just motherhood," you're not alone. Many women walk away from these conversations feeling unheard, confused, and still without answers.

This book is here to change that. You'll find a clear, step-by-step understanding of what's happening beneath the surface—why you feel the way you do, and what you can realistically do about it. You won't find rigid diets or unrealistic wellness routines. Just practical, doable strategies designed for real-life.

Understanding Holistic Health: It's All Connected

As you'll discover throughout this book, the human body operates as a deeply interconnected system where addressing one issue with the power of nutrition and herbal medicine often leads to improvements across multiple areas of health. This holistic perspective underscores a significant limitation of the conventional medical system, which tends to compartmentalize care into specialized silos. For example, a cardiologist focuses on your heart, an ophthalmologist on your eyes, a gastroenterologist on your digestive system, a neurologist on your brain, and an endocrinologist on your hormones. While this specialization allows for advanced expertise, it often overlooks the critical connections between these systems – for example the connection between the gut microbiome and the state of your mental health.

The truth is, no organ or function exists in isolation. Your gut health influences your brain function, your hormone levels impact your cardiovascular health, and even your mental well-being can have profound effects on your immune system. The current siloed approach can miss these essential interdependencies, sometimes addressing symptoms without uncovering the root cause.

This book embraces a whole-body perspective, empowering you to understand and address the underlying factors affecting your health. By adopting this integrative approach, you'll see how small changes in one area – be it diet, lifestyle, or stress management – can ripple outward, creating benefits for your entire well-being.

It is important to note that this guide is not meant to be implemented in full at one time. It is a guide to provide information on issues that are most ailing you over the years.

The Transformative Experience of Motherhood

Becoming a mother is one of the most profound changes a woman can experience. It's not just about taking on a new role – it's a transformation that weaves together the person you were and the person you're becoming. For many, this shift is both exciting and challenging, leaving you to wonder, *who am I now?* This question is both natural and complex. Motherhood doesn't mean leaving behind your past self; it's about integrating the experiences, strengths, and lessons that shape your evolving identity. Yet, the journey is rarely straightforward because you're not just feeling different – you *are* different.

While motherhood brings immense joy and purpose, it can also be physically and emotionally demanding. As mothers, we often find ourselves juggling competing priorities, with our health and well-being falling to the bottom of the list. From the moment you conceive, your body devotes its energy and resources to nurturing new life. Pregnancy, childbirth, and breastfeeding draw heavily on your body's nutrient reserves – the "spark plugs of life" like vitamins and minerals that fuel your energy, immunity, and mental resilience. For many women, especially those with gut health challenges, restoring these depleted stores can take years.

Studies show that 90% of pregnant women in developed countries experience nutrient deficiencies, and these often worsen after birth due to blood loss, breastfeeding, sleepless nights, and the sheer physical demand of caring for a newborn.

Hormonal shifts, sleep deprivation and the physical toll of new motherhood often compound these issues, leaving many mothers feeling exhausted and unwell. When your nutrient levels are sub-optimal, it can impact everything

– from your mood and immune system to your gut health.

On top of that, modern life makes it even harder to stay well. Processed foods, pesticides, environmental toxins, having babies later in life, chronic conditions and stress all challenge our ability to recover and thrive. Without mindful choices – like nourishing ourselves with real food, managing stress, and supporting our gut health – we risk long-term depletion.

This isn't meant to overshadow the beauty of motherhood, but rather to shine a light on the parts we don't often talk about – the hidden struggles of the early years. The seemingly secret woman's business that can almost feel too taboo to talk about openly.

We'll dive into the real, practical steps you can take to uncover the root causes of your exhaustion and start the journey toward reclaiming your energy, vitality, and sense of self. Because sometimes, it's not just about sleep deprivation or adjusting to new responsibilities – it's about addressing deeper health imbalances.

So, with that in mind, let's begin at the start of your motherhood journey and unravel the steps to feeling whole again.

I

Part One

The First Year – When Reality Bites

It's not about doing more or being perfect; it's about understanding what your body truly needs to heal, adapt, and thrive. This section is a gentle but powerful guide to rebuilding your health from the ground up — starting in the fourth trimester (the 3 months after your baby has been earth side) and continuing through your first year as a mother.

1

What is Postnatal Depletion?

It is often said that becoming a mother is the most magical time of your life – when moms are glowing and full of joy, babies are smiling and life is filled with cuddles and soft lullabies. But what if your experience doesn't look like that? What if, instead of feeling overjoyed, you feel exhausted, frazzled, and not quite like yourself?

For so many mothers, the struggle runs deeper than sleepless nights, recovery and adjusting to a new routine. It's more than just being tired – it's a level of depletion that seeps into every part of you. And yet, it's rarely talked about and barely recognized by doctors.

This is postnatal depletion – a deep, long-lasting exhaustion caused by the monumental demands of pregnancy, birth, and motherhood. The symptoms of postnatal depletion can vary from person to person, you might notice it in small ways, such as struggling to concentrate, feeling on edge or overwhelmed and having little to no patience. Or it might feel bigger where you experience constant exhaustion, no matter how much you sleep, digestive issues, unexplained food sensitivities, hair thinning or breakage, persistent anxiety, mood swings and brain fog.

Postnatal depletion can be difficult to recognize because the symptoms vary from person to person, making it challenging to pinpoint, and it is often mistaken for other conditions or simply blamed on what's part and parcel of becoming a mother.

The good news is that this isn't permanent. With the right nourishment, rest, lifestyle changes, health restoration, and support, you can rebuild your strength and reclaim your energy. But first, let's dive deeper into the signs of postnatal depletion, because understanding what's happening in your body is the first step toward recovery.

Isn't this Just the Baby Blues?

It's normal to experience emotional ups and downs after birth. Many mothers go through the "baby blues," which typically start 2 to 3 days postpartum and resolve within a couple of weeks. You might find yourself experiencing mood swings, unexpected crying spells, or trouble sleeping. This is due to not only being sleep deprived and adjusting to a new life but a rapid hormonal shift – during pregnancy, estrogen and progesterone levels are exceptionally high to support your baby's growth. However, within just 24 to 48 hours after birth, these hormones drop drastically, all while you're adjusting to night wakings, physical recovery, a shifting identity, and the demands of a newborn.

Postnatal depletion is different; it lingers. Some women feel it immediately, while others don't recognize it until months or even years later. Instead of temporary hormonal shifts, it's a depletion of essential nutrients and energy that can deeply impact both body and mind.

It is also important to note that postnatal depletion is different to postnatal depression; postnatal depression is a much more serious concern, the differences between them are covered later on in this chapter. If you feel like you're suffering from postnatal depression, it is important to seek help from a trusted health professional to get more support.

The Truth is Recovery Takes Longer than We've Been Told

We often hear about the "fourth trimester" — those early months after birth — as the main window for recovery. But what most mothers aren't told is that true healing and replenishment take much longer. For many, postnatal depletion lingers well beyond the baby stage — long after their child is sleeping through the night, after they've returned to work, or even years later, when symptoms finally become impossible to ignore.

This book explores what happens *after* the fourth trimester — because that's when many women realize just how deeply depleted they've become. If you're still tired, foggy, anxious, or feeling unlike yourself long after those newborn months, you're not broken or failing. You're simply still in need of nourishment, support, and restoration.

The good news is, it's never too late to rebuild your health. With the right tools and understanding, you can begin restoring your energy and vitality — one step at a time.

Recognizing the Signs of Postnatal Depletion

Even years after childbirth, many women find themselves struggling with symptoms they can't quite explain. They push through the exhaustion, brain fog, and emotional ups and downs — often believing this is just part of motherhood. To make things more confusing, postnatal depletion can mimic other health conditions, leaving many wondering if it's simply stress, lack of sleep, or something more.

And while well-meaning friends, family, and even doctors may dismiss these symptoms as "normal," that doesn't make them *healthy*. Common doesn't mean normal, and you don't have to live with it.

Many new mothers experience these challenges early on, but when they persist or intensify over time, it's a clear signal your body needs deeper care. Recognizing these signs is the first step toward true recovery and reclaiming your sense of wellbeing.

(It's important to note that some symptoms may overlap with other health issues. Always consult a qualified health professional to rule out anything more serious.)

Cognitive & Emotional Symptoms

- **Brain Fog:** Difficulty concentrating, memory lapses, trouble focusing, and mental cloudiness. Beyond nutrient deficiencies (iron, B vitamins, omega-3s), brain fog is often linked to poor digestion, low stomach acid, imbalanced gut flora, and disrupted sleep. Integrative medicine also points to underlying stealth infections (like Epstein-Barr Virus or mold exposure) and heavy metal accumulation (such as mercury or copper excess) that impair mitochondrial and neurological function.
- **Depression & Anxiety:** Persistent low moods, excessive worry, or feelings of hopelessness. These can be exacerbated by low serotonin, cortisol dysregulation, blood sugar instability, and omega-3 depletion. Additionally, poor methylation, gut-brain axis dysfunction, or chronic inflammation triggered by stealth pathogens or heavy metal toxicity can further destabilize mood regulation.
- **Mood Swings & Irritability:** Emotional highs and lows that feel out of proportion. In addition to hormonal shifts (especially in estrogen and progesterone), imbalances in zinc, magnesium, and copper can intensify emotional reactivity. Copper excess is particularly relevant postpartum due to estrogen fluctuations and its effect on neurotransmitters.
- **Emotional Numbness:** A sense of disconnection from yourself, your baby, or others. Often rooted in chronic stress, low oxytocin, sleep deprivation, and HPA axis dysfunction. Low vitamin D, poor gut health, and unresolved trauma may also blunt emotional responsiveness.
- **Overwhelm & Easily Stressed:** Feeling drained by everyday tasks. Adrenal fatigue, unstable blood sugar, sleep fragmentation, and nervous system dysregulation all play a role. Histamine intolerance, mold illness, or latent infections (like Lyme or EBV) may also heighten sensitivity to stress.

Energy & Sleep Disturbances

- **Extreme Fatigue:** Exhaustion that persists despite rest. Common drivers include iron and B-vitamin deficiency, mitochondrial dysfunction, low thyroid function, chronic inflammation, and toxin overload (especially from mercury or aluminum). Stealth infections and mold toxicity should also be considered in persistent fatigue.
- **Insomnia or Poor Sleep Quality:** Trouble falling or staying asleep. May stem from magnesium deficiency, blood sugar drops, elevated nighttime cortisol, or overstimulation from caregiving. EMF exposure, mold-related biotoxins, or liver congestion (which peaks detox activity overnight) can also interfere with sleep architecture.
- **Frequent Headaches or Migraines:** Triggers include dehydration, low magnesium, estrogen imbalances, or blood sugar crashes. Heavy metal accumulation (like mercury or aluminum), histamine intolerance, and unresolved stealth infections may also be involved.

Physical & Immune Health

- **Physical Weakness & Muscle Aches:** Often related to low protein, iron, magnesium, and adrenal exhaustion. Mitochondrial fatigue from heavy metal toxicity or chronic viral load may underlie persistent weakness.
- **Dizziness or Lightheadedness:** May be caused by low blood pressure, anemia, adrenal dysregulation, or electrolyte imbalance. POTS (Postural Orthostatic Tachycardia Syndrome) and mold-related illness should be explored in persistent cases.
- **Digestive Issues (Bloating, Constipation, IBS Symptoms):** Pregnancy and birth alter gut bacteria, and postnatal stress can lead to microbiome imbalance, food intolerances, or low stomach acid, which creates the perfect environment for candida overgrowth. Candida can cause bloating, sugar cravings, brain fog, recurrent thrush, rashes, and fatigue. Antibiotic use, hormonal changes, and a high-sugar diet can all contribute to fungal imbalance.

- **Weakened Immune System:** Frequent illness may reflect nutrient depletion, chronic stress, gut dysbiosis, or stealth pathogens. Low stomach acid allows pathogens to bypass the stomach's natural defense barrier.
- **Frequent Infections or Thrush:** Recurrent yeast infections (oral or vaginal thrush) postpartum may be a sign of systemic candida overgrowth, especially if paired with fatigue, brain fog, or bloating. This often stems from antibiotic use, immune suppression, or poor microbial diversity in the gut and vaginal flora.
- **Slow Wound Healing & Easy Bruising:** Indicates impaired collagen production, vitamin C deficiency, or poor protein intake. Zinc, vitamin A, and antioxidant depletion—often from oxidative stress and toxin overload—can delay healing.
- **Dark Circles Under Eyes:** Often due to exhaustion, anemia, liver congestion, food sensitivities, or adrenal dysfunction. Poor lymphatic drainage and histamine overload can also contribute.
- **Joint Pain or Stiffness:** May result from collagen loss, hormonal shifts, or inflammatory responses driven by leaky gut, food intolerances, or mold-related mycotoxins.

Hormonal & Metabolic Changes

- **Unexplained Weight Gain:** Can result from thyroid imbalances, insulin resistance, elevated cortisol, or chronic sleep deprivation. Heavy metals like mercury can interfere with thyroid receptor sensitivity, and gut pathogens can contribute to low-grade systemic inflammation and weight retention.
- **Unusual Food Cravings:** Craving sugar, refined carbs, or yeasty foods may not just reflect blood sugar issues—it can be a hallmark sign of candida overgrowth, which feeds on sugar and manipulates appetite signals. Gut imbalances like candida can also interfere with mineral absorption and immune regulation.
- **Low Libido:** Often linked to estrogen drop, fatigue, and breastfeeding-

related hormonal suppression. Chronic inflammation, low thyroid function, and emotional depletion can further suppress libido.

Hair, Skin, & Dental Health

- **Hair Loss (Beyond Normal Shedding):** Indicates deeper depletion—low iron, zinc, protein, vitamin D, and thyroid dysfunction are common culprits. Copper overload and stealth infections can also disrupt hair growth cycles.
- **Brittle Hair & Nails:** Usually due to low biotin, collagen, or protein malabsorption. Digestive insufficiency, especially from low stomach acid or pancreatic enzymes, may impair nutrient uptake.
- **Dry or Dull Skin:** Caused by dehydration, fatty acid deficiency, and hormonal imbalances. Toxin buildup, oxidative stress, or poor liver function can also reflect through the skin.
- **Premature Aging (Fine Lines, Wrinkles):** Accelerated aging may result from low vitamin C, collagen depletion, and oxidative stress. Heavy metals and stealth infections increase oxidative burden and degrade skin structure.
- **Pale Complexion:** Often signals iron or B12 deficiency, low circulation, or mitochondrial sluggishness.
- **Mouth Ulcers & Gum Sensitivity:** Linked to B2, B12, and C deficiencies. Also, poor gut health, low stomach acid, or viral reactivation (e.g., herpes family viruses) can contribute.
- **Dental Concerns:** Pregnancy depletes calcium, phosphorus, and vitamin D, increasing vulnerability to cavities and enamel erosion. Mouth microbiome imbalance and nutrient absorption issues can exacerbate this.

Other Common Symptoms

- **Heightened Sensitivity to Noise & Overstimulation:** Often due to magnesium deficiency, adrenal fatigue, or nervous system dysregulation. Histamine intolerance, mold, and copper excess can amplify sensory reactivity.
- **Racing Heartbeat (Palpitations):** Can be caused by thyroid shifts, cortisol spikes, electrolyte imbalances, or anxiety. B-vitamin depletion and toxin exposure may impair cardiac function and stress response.
- **Cold Hands & Feet:** Common in thyroid dysfunction, poor circulation, or anemia. Mercury or lead toxicity may also disrupt cellular metabolism and oxygen delivery.
- **Tingling or Numbness in Hands & Feet:** May signal B12 deficiency, poor circulation, or nerve inflammation. Chronic inflammation from stealth infections or mold exposure should be considered in persistent cases.

Understanding the Causes of Postnatal Depletion

In a nutshell, motherhood draws deeply from every part of you — your body, your emotions, and your nutritional reserves. Growing, birthing, and nourishing a baby places extraordinary demands on your system. When combined with sub-optimal gut health, pre-existing nutritional deficiencies, new responsibilities, hormone imbalances, stealth infections, the toxicities of modern living, or sleep deprivation, it can feel overwhelming.

For many women, the postpartum period is like navigating a perfect storm — a convergence of physical exhaustion, emotional upheaval, and societal pressures that leave them depleted and stretched thin. Postnatal depletion isn't just "feeling tired." It is the result of the immense physiological, emotional, and psychological toll of pregnancy, childbirth, and early motherhood. By understanding the key contributors to this state, mothers and their support networks can take meaningful steps toward recovery and renewal.

To truly support new mothers, it's essential to recognize the multifaceted causes of postnatal depletion. This section explores the physical, emotional, psychological, and societal factors that contribute to this condition, shedding light on why so many mothers struggle and offering insights into the path to recovery.

1. The Emotional Load of New Motherhood

Motherhood brings with it a wave of new responsibilities, many of which can feel relentless. Caring for a newborn demands constant attention, with interrupted sleep and the round-the-clock feeding and soothing often leaving mothers physically and emotionally drained.

For many, this is compounded by a fear of inadequacy – feeling the weight of societal expectations to be the "perfect" parent. The pressure to "have it all together" often fosters self-doubt, leading mothers to question their abilities and worth. If a woman has a history of anxiety or depression, these feelings may intensify, creating a cycle of emotional exhaustion that's hard to break.

Adding to this burden is the reality of social isolation. With the demands of childcare, many mothers find their social lives shrinking, leaving them lonely and without the vital support networks that could ease the transition into motherhood. For those balancing work with parenting, the struggle to maintain a sense of professional identity while meeting the needs of a newborn can feel like an impossible juggling act.

2. Nutritional Depletion: A Hidden Epidemic

Pregnancy, childbirth, and breastfeeding place extraordinary demands on a mother's body, rapidly depleting essential nutrients. While the focus often shifts entirely to the baby's needs, the mother's own nutritional health can be overlooked.

Breastfeeding alone requires a significant increase in nutrients like calcium, iron, and essential fatty acids. Yet, in the whirlwind of new motherhood, many women rely on quick, processed meals or skip meals altogether, compounding nutrient deficiencies. Sleep deprivation and stress only worsen the situation, often disrupting gut health and reducing the body's ability to absorb and utilize nutrients.

These deficiencies manifest in exhaustion, irritability, and feelings of emotional instability – symptoms many mothers mistakenly accept as "just part of the process."

3. The Roller-Coaster of Hormonal Changes

After childbirth, the body undergoes dramatic hormonal shifts that can profoundly affect a mother's mood, energy levels, and overall well-being. Hormones like estrogen and progesterone, which surged during pregnancy, plummet post-delivery, often leaving women feeling emotionally unstable and physically drained.

For some, postpartum thyroiditis – an inflammation of the thyroid – further disrupts energy levels and mood, while the ongoing production of cortisol, the stress hormone, strains the adrenal glands. This hormonal roller-coaster not only affects emotional balance but also amplifies physical exhaustion, leaving many mothers feeling like they're running on empty.

4. Gut Health and the Microbiome

Gut health plays a critical, though often overlooked, role in postpartum recovery. The gut microbiome – the delicate balance of bacteria and microorganisms in the digestive system – can be disrupted during pregnancy and childbirth. Antibiotics given in the drip (often unknowingly to the mother) during labor, dietary changes caused by morning sickness, stress, and stress all contribute to imbalances that affect digestion, nutrient absorption, and even hormonal regulation.

When gut health is compromised, the effects ripple through the body, leading to chronic inflammation, poor nutrient uptake, and a weakened immune system – all of which deepen the sense of depletion.

5. Stealth Underlying Chronic Infections: The Silent Energy Drain

Underlying infections, whether bacterial, viral, or fungal, can silently sap energy reserves. After childbirth, a mother's immune system is already stretched thin, making it harder to fight off infections that may have been dormant. These infections can go unnoticed, yet they add to the fatigue and hinder the recovery process.

6. Sleep Deprivation

Sleep deprivation is often the most visible – and yet underestimated – contributor to postnatal depletion. Interrupted sleep, whether due to night feedings or the constant vigilance required for newborn care, prevents the body from entering the deep, restorative phases of rest.

Over time, this chronic lack of sleep diminishes cognitive function, weakens the immune system, and exacerbates hormonal imbalances and nutrient deficiencies. It's no wonder so many mothers feel as though they're running on fumes, stuck in a cycle of exhaustion that seems impossible to break.

The Perfect Storm

Each of these factors – emotional strain, nutrient deficiencies, hormonal fluctuations, gut health disruptions, infections, and sleep deprivation - interacts to create a perfect storm of postnatal depletion. Together, they drain a mother's physical and emotional reserves, leaving her feeling trapped in a cycle of fatigue, irritability, and overwhelm.

But there is hope. By understanding the interconnected nature of these challenges, mothers can take the first steps toward reclaiming their health and vitality. With awareness and the right tools, mothers can navigate through the storm and emerge stronger, ready to embrace the transformative journey of motherhood with renewed energy and joy.

Why Modern-Day Mothers Are More at Risk

Modern motherhood isn't what it used to be. Today's mothers are navigating a perfect storm of stressors that previous generations didn't face—at least not all at once. While motherhood has always been demanding, the landscape has shifted in ways that make physical recovery, emotional resilience, and long-term well-being harder to maintain.

We're having children later in life, often while balancing demanding careers, running households, and living under social pressure to "bounce back" quickly after birth. But it's not just our lifestyle that's changed—our internal biology is also being impacted by factors our mothers and grandmothers never had to contend with.

More Toxins, Less Resilience

Today's women are exposed to thousands of synthetic chemicals that simply didn't exist a few generations ago. These include endocrine-disrupting compounds in plastics and personal care products, pesticides on our food, and heavy metals in our water supply. Research shows that even low levels of chronic exposure to these toxins can interfere with hormone balance, fertility, metabolism, and postpartum recovery.

A Gut Out of Balance

The health of your gut is fundamental to your overall vitality—but modern life doesn't support a thriving microbiome. Compared to our ancestors, our diets today contain fewer whole foods and more ultra-processed options, sugar, additives, and antibiotics (both prescribed and hidden in the food supply). This leads to **gut dysbiosis**—an imbalance in the microbial community that affects digestion, nutrient absorption, immunity, and even mood.

An imbalanced gut can mean that even when you *do* eat well, your body struggles to absorb the nutrients it desperately needs. This is especially critical postpartum, when nutrient demands are at their highest (restoring gut health is covered extensively in chapter 4 and chapter 15).

Pregnancy at an Older Age

The average age of first-time motherhood has steadily risen across the developed world. In countries like Australia and the UK, it's now over 30, with a growing number of women having babies in their late 30s or early 40s.

While there's nothing wrong with starting a family later, it's important to recognize the physiological reality: the body doesn't recover as efficiently with age. Hormone levels decline, tissue repair slows, and the body's stress response becomes more reactive. What may have been an easy recovery in your early 20s often feels far more depleting a decade or two later.

But Is It Really Worse Than Before?

Some skeptics might ask, "Didn't women always go through this?" And yes—childbirth has always been a major physiological event. But here's what's different now:

- **We're more depleted before pregnancy even starts**, thanks to chronic stress, sleep deprivation, and poor dietary quality.
- **We're under more pressure to 'do it all'**—with less communal support and more individual responsibility.
- **We're exposed to more environmental and emotional stressors**, while our recovery time is often shorter and unsupported.

In the past, mothers typically had more help, lived in extended families or close-knit communities, and weren't expected to return to work within weeks of giving birth. Today, many mothers don't get that same village—and their bodies bear the brunt of it.

Here's What the Research Shows

- **Environmental toxins impact maternal health:** Endocrine disruptors (found in plastics, pesticides, and skincare) are linked to fertility issues, hormone imbalance, and impaired postpartum recovery.
- **Gut dysbiosis slows healing:** Disruption of the gut microbiome is associated with inflammation, anxiety, fatigue, and poor nutrient absorption after birth.
- **Older mothers face more challenges:** Women over 35 are more likely to experience adrenal fatigue, thyroid issues, and slower recovery from iron and nutrient loss.
- **50% of mothers feel exhausted for years after giving birth:** Many assume it's just part of motherhood—but it doesn't have to be.
- **Iron deficiency affects up to 40% of postpartum women:** Especially those over 35, whose iron stores take longer to rebuild.
- **Bone loss is real:** Mothers lose up to 5% of their bone density with each pregnancy if calcium, vitamin D, and magnesium are not restored.
- **Mental health risks are rising:** In Australia, nearly 1 in 5 women report perinatal depression or anxiety, with studies showing that maternal depletion is a major contributing factor.

What This Means for Modern Mothers

Recognizing that your body is under more pressure than ever isn't about scaring you; it's about empowering you to take action. When we understand the unique stressors affecting modern mothers, we can stop blaming ourselves for not "bouncing back" and start giving our bodies what they actually need.

With the right support—nutritional, emotional, and environmental—postnatal recovery doesn't have to be a silent struggle. The more we listen to our bodies and nourish them intentionally, the stronger, clearer, and more resilient we become—not just for our children, but for ourselves.

Why Addressing Postnatal Depletion is Important

If you've got multiple signs of postnatal depletion as outlined above, this is your body waving a red flag that it needs support. Postnatal depletion is real, and if left unchecked, you could find yourself running on empty for far longer than necessary.

Ignoring it won't just make today harder; it sets the stage for long-term struggles. Without proper intervention, your health could continue to decline, leaving you with low energy, a foggy brain, and a body that's more prone to illness. When you're too sluggish to chase your dreams and too run-down to enjoy life's moments, everything feels like an uphill battle.

Chances are, if you've been feeling off for a while, there's more than one issue at play. Postnatal depletion can involve a cocktail of nutrient deficiencies, poor gut health, adrenal fatigue, hormone imbalances, and thyroid issues. It's not just one thing, and fixing it requires more than a quick fix.

If you've been struggling with nagging health problems for years, it's important to remember that healing takes time. Unwinding the damage and bringing your body back to a balanced state – homeostasis – often calls for a multifaceted approach. It's not just about changing your diet, although nutrition is arguably the cornerstone of recovery. Optimal nutrition provides your body with the high-quality building blocks it needs to produce hormones, neurotransmitters, and energy, and to repair and heal.

But that's not all. Healing postnatal depletion also means shifting your mindset, improving your gut health, and making key lifestyle adjustments. This guide gives you a step-by-step, actionable plan – not just for recovering from postnatal depletion, but for living a happier, healthier life.

Postnatal Depletion vs. Postnatal Depression: Key Differences

While postnatal depletion and postnatal depression (PND) can share some overlapping symptoms, they are distinct conditions that require different approaches to treatment and understanding. It is essential to recognize the differences between them, even though both can significantly impact a new mother's health and well-being.

Postnatal depletion is largely a physical issue related to nutrient deficiencies and energy reserves, while postnatal depression is a mental health condition that requires psychological support. Understanding this distinction is crucial for proper diagnosis and treatment. Mothers experiencing either condition should seek professional help, whether it be through dietary changes, supplementation, or mental health counseling, to restore both physical and emotional well-being.

Postnatal Depression: A Mental Health Condition

Postnatal depression (PND) is a significant mental health condition that occurs after childbirth, affecting approximately 10-15% of new mothers. PND goes beyond feelings of tiredness or low energy; it is marked by persistent sadness, hopelessness, anxiety, and difficulties in bonding with the baby. Mothers with PND often experience changes in sleeping and eating patterns, as well as an overwhelming sense of inadequacy or guilt.

Symptoms of postnatal depression are more significant than postnatal depletion and may include:

- Persistent sadness or low mood
- Loss of interest in activities that were once enjoyable
- Feelings of guilt, hopelessness, or worthlessness
- Difficulty bonding with the baby
- Disrupted sleep and appetite

- Ongoing unexplained anger, anxiety, crying or panic attacks
- In some cases, thoughts of self-harm or harm to the baby

While postnatal depletion is primarily physical in nature, PND is a mental health issue that often requires psychological intervention, counseling, and sometimes medication. Importantly, while postnatal depression has many causes – ranging from hormonal shifts to psychological stressors – nutrient deficiencies can exacerbate the condition.

Overlapping Symptoms and the Importance of Differentiation

There can be a crossover of symptoms between postnatal depletion and postnatal depression, such as fatigue, irritability, and trouble focusing. Nutritional deficiencies commonly seen in postnatal depletion, such as low omega-3 fatty acids and vitamin D, have been linked to a higher risk of developing postnatal depression. However, it is critical to distinguish between the two.

Postnatal depletion is more about nutrient and energy recovery, whereas postnatal depression is rooted in deeper emotional and mental health issues. Addressing postnatal depletion with adequate nutrition, rest, and lifestyle adjustments can often improve a mother's sense of well-being. But postnatal depression requires specific mental health interventions to address emotional distress and ensure the mother can bond with her baby and recover fully.

The Role of Nutrients in Postnatal Depression

Recent research has highlighted the role of nutrient deficiencies in postnatal depression, particularly deficiencies in omega-3 fatty acids and vitamin D. Both of these nutrients play essential roles in brain function and mood regulation. Omega-3, specifically DHA, are crucial for reducing inflammation and supporting brain health, while vitamin D helps regulate mood and immune function.

A deficiency in these nutrients, which is common in many postpartum women, can exacerbate feelings of depression, anxiety, and emotional instability. This underscores the importance of addressing nutritional gaps as part of the treatment plan for postnatal depression. In some cases, replenishing these nutrients can alleviate symptoms and improve mood, though PND typically requires more comprehensive psychological care.

Recovering from Postnatal Depletion

Recovering from postnatal depletion is a journey, not a quick fix. It's not something that can be solved with one magic pill, or even a few full nights of sleep again. While these things can certainly help, true healing comes from a more holistic approach - one that nurtures both your body and mind.

As you take the steps outlined in this book, you won't just be climbing out of the exhaustion - you'll be rebuilding your strength from the inside out. You'll be restoring your gut health, replenishing vital nutrients, balancing your blood sugar, recharging your energy, and supporting your hormones - all essential for feeling like yourself again.

2

The Postpartum Hormonal Roller-Coaster

The postpartum period brings one of the fastest and most dramatic shifts in hormone levels that a woman will ever experience. Within 24 hours of giving birth, estrogen and progesterone levels plummet, creating a hormonal change more rapid than puberty or menopause. At the same time, hormones like oxytocin and prolactin rise to support bonding and breastfeeding. These fluctuations can bring emotional highs and lows, energy crashes and unexpected physical changes – all of which are a normal part of recovery.

Understanding what your body is going through can help you embrace this unique time with a little more peace and patience. By recognizing the natural ebb and flow of postpartum hormones, you can support your recovery holistically, allowing your body to heal while nurturing your well-being.

After childbirth, your body is in rapid transition, adapting to a non-pregnant state while also supporting lactation, healing, and the demands of early motherhood.

1. **Estrogen and Progesterone Crash:** Estrogen and progesterone were at peak levels during pregnancy, helping to support the baby's growth and your own physical adjustments. But after delivery, they drop sharply and return to pre-pregnancy levels within just 24 hours. This sudden dip is linked with mood changes, low energy, and even hair loss, leaving

many mothers feeling more emotional than usual.

2. **Oxytocin the Bonding Hormone:** Oxytocin, often called the "love hormone," is essential for uterine contraction and helps control bleeding after birth. Levels rise as you hold or breastfeed your baby, fostering that special bond between mother and child. Breastfeeding also helps increase oxytocin, which may reduce anxiety and strengthen emotional resilience.

3. **Prolactin the Milk-Making Hormone:** Prolactin levels increase with breastfeeding, signaling milk production and helping you stay focused on your baby's needs. It also has a calming effect, though it can reduce energy levels, which may explain the natural pull many mothers feel toward nesting and spending time close to their baby.

4. **Cortisol and Stress Response:** Cortisol, a stress hormone, tends to be higher after birth as your body remains on alert to respond to your newborn's needs. While it aids in alertness, elevated cortisol can sometimes heighten anxiety. Finding ways to soothe yourself is key to managing cortisol levels.

Signs Your Hormones Need Support After the 4th Trimester

After giving birth, your body undergoes a powerful hormonal recalibration. The sharp drop in estrogen and progesterone—combined with fluctuations in oxytocin, prolactin, cortisol, and thyroid hormones—affects far more than your reproductive system. These hormonal shifts influence your brain, energy, mood, and physical well-being.

And while much of the focus is placed on recovery during the first 12 weeks postpartum—the "fourth trimester"—for many women, hormonal imbalance can persist for months or even years, especially when ongoing sleep deprivation, nutrient depletion and stress are present. Recognizing the signs that your hormones may still be out of balance is the first step toward healing and reclaiming your vitality.

1. Emotional Sensitivity and Mood Swings

Emotional ups and downs are expected in early postpartum, but when they continue long after the newborn phase, it could indicate ongoing hormonal instability.

- Estrogen supports serotonin, your brain's "feel-good" neurotransmitter. When estrogen remains low, serotonin levels may also stay low—leading to tearfulness, irritability, or apathy.
- Progesterone has a natural calming effect. Its continued deficiency may leave you feeling anxious, edgy, or easily overwhelmed.

These symptoms may linger well beyond the initial adjustment period, signaling a need for hormonal and nervous system support.

2. Anxiety and Heightened Stress Response

Persistent anxiety, racing thoughts, or a sense of being constantly "on edge" may reflect an imbalance in cortisol, the body's primary stress hormone.

- Prolonged sleep deprivation, emotional load, and overstimulation from constant caregiving can keep cortisol elevated, taxing your adrenal system.
- Oxytocin, the bonding and calming hormone, may also fluctuate depending on breastfeeding experiences, touch, and emotional safety—impacting how supported or emotionally grounded you feel.

If the smallest things tip you into overwhelm or you can't seem to wind down, your stress response may be stuck in overdrive.

3. Fatigue That Doesn't Improve with Rest

Exhaustion is expected with young children—but when fatigue becomes unrelenting, even after a full night's sleep or a restful weekend, deeper hormonal drivers may be at play.

- Low estrogen slows energy metabolism and contributes to lethargy.
- Postpartum thyroiditis (inflammation of the thyroid) can cause fatigue, brain fog, mood changes, and unexplained weight shifts.
- High prolactin levels, often elevated during breastfeeding, can have a sedative effect that contributes to mental and physical exhaustion.

If you're tired to your bones, despite rest and caffeine, it's time to look beyond lifestyle.

4. Physical Symptoms: Night Sweats, Hair Loss, Breast Changes

Hormonal shifts can affect your entire body, not just your emotions.

- **Night Sweats & Hot Flashes**: Declining estrogen disrupts temperature regulation. These symptoms can continue for many months after childbirth, especially during weaning or hormonal transition.
- **Hair Loss**: Postpartum hair shedding typically peaks around 3–4 months but may persist if estrogen remains low or nutrient stores aren't rebuilt.
- **Breast Changes**: Even after weaning, breast tenderness, swelling, or softness may occur due to hormonal fluctuations or rebalancing.

While these changes are common, if they linger or worsen, they may reflect unresolved hormonal or nutritional imbalances.

5. "Mommy Brain" and Mental Fog

If you often forget words mid-sentence, misplace items, or feel like your brain is running through mud, you're not imagining it.

- Estrogen influences neurotransmitters like dopamine and serotonin—critical for memory, attention, and cognition.
- Chronic cortisol elevation (from stress and broken sleep) impairs memory formation and executive function.
- Low thyroid function also contributes to slowed thinking and difficulty concentrating.

Mental clarity often improves with proper nourishment and sleep, but lasting fog can point to hormonal or adrenal depletion.

6. Low Libido and Physical Discomfort

Reduced interest in intimacy is very common, but when it doesn't naturally return—or is accompanied by discomfort—it deserves attention.

- Low estrogen may cause vaginal dryness, thinning tissues, and discomfort during sex.
- Elevated prolactin (especially while breastfeeding) suppresses libido to prioritize caretaking over reproduction.
- Emotional overload, changes in body image, and lack of time or privacy can compound physical issues, further diminishing desire.

Reconnecting with your body and sense of self often starts with supporting hormonal recovery and creating emotional safety.

7. Long-Term Mood Challenges

When low mood persists well beyond the first few months—or intensifies over time—it may signal deeper imbalances.

- The steep drop in estrogen and progesterone after birth can trigger mood instability in sensitive individuals.
- Thyroid dysfunction, chronic inflammation, and key nutrient deficiencies (iron, B12, omega-3s, zinc) can also contribute to long-term depression and emotional disconnection.
- Some women don't experience postpartum depression until 6–12 months later, especially during weaning or return to work.

You don't need a formal diagnosis to take these symptoms seriously. Low mood and emotional numbness can be real signs that your body and brain need replenishment—not judgment.

Recovery Takes Time—And Support

Contrary to cultural expectations, hormone balance doesn't bounce back six weeks after birth. For many women, it can take a full year or more to restore hormonal resilience—especially without rest, nutrient-dense food, or support.

These symptoms aren't just "part of being a mum." They're important messages from your body, letting you know it's time to replenish what's been lost.

Healing is possible. And it begins by listening to your body, honoring its needs, and giving yourself permission to heal—well beyond the fourth trimester.

Hormone Fluctuations and Underlying Health Conditions in Postpartum

It is entirely normal for mothers to experience significant hormonal fluctuations during pregnancy and the postpartum period. These changes are a natural part of the body adapting to pregnancy, childbirth, and lactation. However, for many women, the postpartum period also exacerbates underlying hormone-related conditions that may have gone unnoticed prior to pregnancy. Conditions such as hypothyroidism, polycystic ovary syndrome (PCOS) and adrenal dysfunction can become more pronounced, compounding the challenges of recovery and adaptation during this demanding phase of life.

The hormonal shifts after childbirth are dramatic, with estrogen and progesterone levels plummeting to pre-pregnancy levels within days. Prolactin levels rise to support breastfeeding, while cortisol, often elevated during pregnancy, fluctuates in response to stress and sleep deprivation. These changes are normal but can worsen pre-existing imbalances, leading to symptoms such as persistent fatigue, mood swings, weight retention, hair loss, and brain fog. For example, studies indicate that as many as 23% of postpartum women experience hypothyroidism, which can cause extreme tiredness and depression if untreated.

Hormonal imbalances during this period can also make mental health challenges more difficult to manage. Postpartum depression (PPD) affects approximately 1 in 7 women, with hormonal instability being a significant contributing factor according to the American College of Obstetricians and Gynecologists. Low thyroid function, blood sugar dysregulation, and adrenal fatigue can all mimic or intensify symptoms of PPD, making it essential to identify and address these issues early.

Additionally, the postpartum period often unmasks symptoms of PCOS, which affects 6-12% of women of reproductive age according to the Centers for Disease Control and Prevention. These symptoms, including irregular periods, weight gain, and insulin resistance, can interfere with recovery and a mother's ability to feel like herself again. Combined with the stress of caring for a newborn, unresolved hormonal imbalances may lead to a vicious cycle of exhaustion, poor self-care, and worsening symptoms.

Acknowledging and addressing these underlying conditions is crucial for a smoother postpartum recovery. Hormone-specific blood tests, thyroid panels, and functional medicine approaches like adrenal and nutrient support can be powerful tools to identify imbalances and guide interventions. Early intervention not only helps mothers feel more like themselves but also supports their ability to care for their growing families.

Natural Ways to Restore Hormonal Balance

Hormones are the body's chemical messengers, influencing metabolism, mood, energy levels, and reproductive health. After birth, the body undergoes a profound hormonal shift, which can leave many mothers feeling depleted, emotional, or overwhelmed. From a holistic nutritionist's perspective, here's how to naturally restore balance and support your well-being during the postpartum period.

Nourish Your Body with Hormone-Supportive Foods

Food is the foundation of hormonal health. Nutrient-dense whole foods provide the building blocks for hormone production, neurotransmitter function, and cellular repair.

- **Healthy Fats**: Hormones are made from cholesterol and healthy fats, meaning adequate fat intake is essential for postpartum recovery. Sources like avocados, extra virgin olive oil, fatty fish, coconut, nuts, and seeds provide essential fatty acids that support estrogen, progesterone, and cortisol regulation. Omega-3 fats, particularly DHA from wild-caught salmon and sardines, also reduce postpartum inflammation and support brain function.

- **Protein-Rich Foods**: Protein is necessary for tissue repair, enzyme production, and hormone synthesis. High-quality protein sources like pasture-raised eggs, grass-fed meats, wild-caught fish, and collagen-rich bone broths help rebuild and restore postpartum tissues while stabilizing satiety hormones and blood sugar, which directly affects insulin and cortisol levels.
- **Complex Carbohydrates**: The right carbohydrates provide sustained energy and help manage stress hormones. Fiber-rich options like sweet potatoes, quinoa, legumes, and whole grains prevent blood sugar crashes and support serotonin production—our "feel-good" hormone that often dips postpartum.
- **Mineral-Rich Foods**: Zinc (from oysters, pumpkin seeds, and beef) is essential for immune function and hormone balance, particularly progesterone. Magnesium (from leafy greens, dark chocolate, and almonds) relaxes the nervous system, improves sleep, and supports adrenal health. Selenium (from Brazil nuts) is critical for thyroid hormone production, which often takes a hit postpartum.

Support Blood Sugar Balance

Balanced blood sugar is crucial for postpartum recovery, as insulin fluctuations can contribute to fatigue, mood swings, and sugar cravings. When blood sugar spikes and crashes, cortisol (the stress hormone) is overproduced, leading to further hormonal imbalances.

- **Eat Protein and Fat at Each Meal**: These macronutrients slow glucose absorption, preventing insulin spikes and crashes that can trigger anxiety and fatigue. Pair carbohydrates with protein to maintain energy and mood stability.
- **Eat Regularly**: Skipping meals or going too long without eating can increase stress hormones, making it harder for the body to recover. Aim for three balanced meals a day with small, protein-rich snacks if needed.
- **Reduce Processed Sugar and Refined Carbohydrates**: Highly processed

foods cause rapid blood sugar fluctuations, exacerbating postpartum depletion and hormone dysregulation. Instead, choose natural sources of sweetness like berries, dates, or dark chocolate.

Optimize Gut Health

A healthy gut is essential for breaking down and eliminating excess hormones, reducing inflammation, and absorbing nutrients necessary for postpartum healing. The gut microbiome also influences estrogen metabolism and serotonin production.

- **Consume Probiotic-Rich Foods**: Fermented foods like kefir, yogurt, sauerkraut, and kimchi introduce beneficial bacteria that support digestion and hormone balance. These bacteria help regulate estrogen metabolism in the gut, reducing symptoms of estrogen dominance.
- **Eat Fiber-Rich Foods**: Flaxseeds, chia seeds, vegetables, and legumes act as prebiotics, feeding good gut bacteria and promoting regular bowel movements. Regular elimination is essential for detoxifying excess estrogen and preventing its reabsorption.
- **Reduce Gut Irritants**: Processed foods, artificial sweeteners, and seed oils can trigger inflammation and gut dysbiosis, further disrupting hormonal balance. Focus on whole, unprocessed foods to support a healthy microbiome.

Prioritize Restorative Sleep

Poor sleep increases cortisol and depletes progesterone, worsening postpartum mood imbalances, anxiety, and fatigue. Sleep is when the body restores hormone levels, repairs tissues, and balances the nervous system.

- **Nap When Possible**: Even short naps can help counteract sleep deprivation and reduce cortisol buildup.
- **Create a Sleep-Friendly Routine**: Winding down with herbal teas (like

chamomile or passionflower), magnesium baths, and minimizing screen exposure before bed can help improve sleep quality.
- **Ask for Help**: New mothers often try to do everything themselves, but even small breaks facilitated by a partner or support system can make a difference.

Reduce Stress and Support the Nervous System

Chronic stress leads to excess cortisol production, which depletes progesterone and suppresses thyroid function – two common hormonal imbalances postpartum. Managing stress helps restore balance to these key hormones.

- **Practice Deep Breathing or Meditation**: Slow, intentional breathing activates the parasympathetic nervous system (the body's "rest and digest" mode), reducing stress hormone levels.
- **Use Adaptogenic Herbs**: Herbs like ashwagandha and holy basil help the body adapt to stress, supporting adrenal function. However, consult a healthcare provider before introducing herbal supplements.
- **Engage in Gentle Movement**: Light stretching, yoga, or walking in nature can lower cortisol, improve circulation, and boost mood-enhancing endorphins.

Replenish Essential Nutrients

Pregnancy and childbirth deplete key vitamins and minerals, making postpartum replenishment essential for restoring hormonal equilibrium.

- **Iron**: Low iron levels contribute to fatigue, brain fog, and poor oxygen transport. Grass-fed beef, liver, and leafy greens are excellent sources. Pair with vitamin C-rich foods (like citrus or bell peppers) for better absorption.
- **B Vitamins**: These support neurotransmitter function, energy metabolism, and stress resilience. Sources include eggs, liver, whole

grains, and leafy greens.
- **Vitamin D**: Essential for immune health, mood regulation, and calcium absorption. Sunlight exposure and fatty fish such as salmon provide natural sources, but supplementation may be needed.
- **Choline**: Important for brain function, memory, and hormone production. Found in eggs, liver, and salmon.
- **Omega-3**: Reduce postpartum inflammation, support brain function, and balance prostaglandins, which regulate hormones. Found in fatty fish, flaxseeds, and walnuts.

Support Progesterone Production

After childbirth, a woman's body undergoes rapid hormonal adjustments, one of the most notable being the steep drop in progesterone. Often referred to as the "pregnancy hormone," progesterone plays an essential role in maintaining pregnancy and supporting mental and physical well-being. Its decline postpartum is normal, yet when levels fall too low or remain imbalanced, women can experience significant mood changes, sleep disturbances, and even postpartum depression. Holistic nutrition, which focuses on whole, nutrient-dense foods, can offer effective ways to support hormonal health and balance, particularly by encouraging the body's natural production of progesterone.

Progesterone is produced by the ovaries and the adrenal glands, playing a vital role in regulating the menstrual cycle, supporting pregnancy, and impacting mood. During pregnancy, progesterone levels increase significantly to support the developing fetus and prepare the body for childbirth. After birth, however, these levels drop rapidly as the placenta, which produces large amounts of progesterone, is no longer present. This shift is one of the sharpest hormonal changes that occurs, which can contribute to the mood instability many new mothers experience. Research suggests that up to 20% of postpartum women may experience some form of mood disorder, with hormonal shifts being a significant factor.

Holistic nutrition emphasizes nutrient-dense foods that can naturally support hormonal balance, targeting the adrenal glands and ovaries, which continue to produce progesterone after pregnancy.

Consuming foods rich in vitamin B6, magnesium, zinc, and healthy fats helps support these endocrine functions and maintains stable hormone levels.

1. Vitamin B6: A Key Nutrient for Progesterone Production

Vitamin B6 plays an important role in progesterone production, as it acts as a co-factor for enzymes involved in hormone synthesis. Studies have shown that higher B6 intake is associated with improved progesterone levels, especially in those experiencing hormonal imbalances. **Foods rich in vitamin B6 include poultry, eggs, sweet potatoes, and bananas**, which can easily be incorporated into a postpartum diet.

2. Magnesium: Essential for Adrenal Health and Stress Reduction

Magnesium is essential for adrenal health, which is closely linked to hormonal stability and progesterone levels. Magnesium deficiencies can exacerbate stress responses, causing the body to overproduce cortisol at the expense of progesterone. **Dark leafy greens, nuts, seeds, and legumes are rich in magnesium** and can support both mental well-being and hormonal health. In fact, research suggests that magnesium supplementation can improve sleep and reduce anxiety in postpartum women, both of which are important for hormone regulation.

3. Zinc: Boosting Ovarian Health and Progesterone Production

Zinc is an important mineral for reproductive health, supporting ovarian function and helping maintain balanced hormone production. Zinc deficiencies have been linked to lower progesterone levels, which can worsen postpartum mood disturbances. **Including foods like pumpkin seeds, lentils, beef, and seafood can help increase zinc intake naturally.**

4. Healthy Fats: Building Blocks for Progesterone and Other Hormones

Hormones, including progesterone, are synthesized from cholesterol and other fats. A diet low in healthy fats can impair hormone production, leading to imbalances. Consuming foods rich in healthy fats, such as avocados, olive oil, nuts, and fatty fish, provides the necessary components for the body to produce hormones effectively. Omega-3 fatty acids, found in fish such as salmon and mackerel, have also been shown to have anti-inflammatory effects, supporting overall endocrine health.

Gentle Detoxification and Hormone Clearance

Your liver plays a key role in metabolizing and clearing excess hormones from the body. Supporting liver function is essential for maintaining hormonal balance and reducing the risk of issues like estrogen dominance. In the first year after birth — especially while breastfeeding — it's important to focus on gentle, supportive detoxification rather than intense or restrictive methods.

More comprehensive detox strategies will be shared later in this book, but for now, here are the safest and most effective ways to support your body in the early postpartum period:

- **Stay Hydrated:** Drinking plenty of water helps your liver and kidneys flush out excess hormones. Opt for filtered water with a squeeze of lemon to gently support liver function.
- **Eat Liver-Supportive Foods:** Include foods that naturally enhance liver detoxification, such as dandelion tea, beets, cruciferous vegetables (like broccoli, Brussels sprouts, and cabbage), and turmeric.
- **Support Natural Detox Pathways:** Gentle movement that encourages sweating, Epsom salt baths, and dry brushing can help stimulate lymphatic flow and promote the elimination of toxins.

Connect and Seek Support

Emotional well-being is a vital — and often underestimated — factor in hormonal balance. When we feel isolated, overwhelmed, or unsupported, the body tends to stay in a prolonged state of stress. This triggers the release of cortisol, the body's primary stress hormone, which plays a major role in energy, sleep, digestion, and inflammation.

In small, short-term amounts, cortisol is helpful. But when it remains elevated due to chronic emotional stress or lack of support, it can disrupt the delicate balance of other hormones — especially progesterone, estrogen, insulin, and thyroid hormones. High cortisol can also make it harder to sleep, lower your resilience, and increase feelings of anxiety, depletion, and burnout.

That's why connection matters. Positive social interaction helps reduce cortisol levels and encourages the release of calming, feel-good hormones like oxytocin, which supports nervous system regulation and emotional healing. Even small moments of connection — a supportive conversation, being heard without judgment, feeling seen by a partner or friend — can help your body shift out of survival mode and into a state where real healing and hormonal balance can occur.

In a season of life that can feel isolating, consider the following ways to support your emotional well-being:

- **Surround Yourself with Supportive People**: Whether it's a partner, friends, or a postpartum support or mother's group, having a strong network can significantly impact mental and emotional health.
- **Practice Self-Care**: Even small acts of self-care, like journaling, reading, or a short walk outside, can provide stress relief and emotional balance.
- **Seek Professional Guidance When Needed**: If symptoms persist, working with a qualified practitioner can help identify deeper hormonal imbalances and tailor an approach specific to your needs.

3

Nutritional Replenishment and the Impact of Vitamin and Mineral Deficiencies

Pregnancy and childbirth place extraordinary demands on the body - but the postpartum period can be just as taxing, physically, mentally, and emotionally. Recovery isn't just about getting more rest; it's about deep replenishment. Nutrition is one of the most powerful tools a mother has to restore energy, support healing, and rebuild her overall well-being.

Yet, the reality is striking: even in high-income countries, up to 90% of pregnant women are malnourished. Studies from the UK, New Zealand, and Singapore reveal widespread deficiencies in essential nutrients like vitamin B12, vitamin D, folate, riboflavin, and B6. Many women begin motherhood already depleted - and it's no surprise that postpartum recovery often feels like an uphill battle.

Even when a mother has access to plenty of food and follows mainstream dietary guidelines, nutritional depletion can persist. This issue is often overlooked, despite how clearly women *feel* its effects: constant fatigue, mood changes, poor memory, and a sense that something just isn't right.

A combination of modern dietary habits, poor gut health, and the immense physiological demands of pregnancy, breastfeeding, and postpartum life all contribute to the depletion of key nutrients. Deficiencies in iron, vitamin

D, b vitamins, omega-3 and other nutrients - which are already common before pregnancy - can deepen during this time, impacting energy levels, mood, immune function and hormone balance. Left unaddressed, these gaps may lead to long-term issues like anemia, bone loss, and mood issues.

Mothers give so much of themselves, not just their love, time, care but their own nutrient stores from their bones and tissues and energy. Growing a baby from scratch is a miraculous achievement, but it comes at a cost. That's why many mothers feel fundamentally different after birth: older, more exhausted, less resilient. While it's easy to blame these changes on sleep deprivation or the chaos of early motherhood, the deeper truth is that much of this shift is rooted in nutritional depletion.

Thoughtful, targeted nourishment lays the foundation not just for short-term recovery, but for long-term vitality and well-being.

Why Nutrient Deficiencies Are the New Normal

Nutrient deficiencies, particularly mineral deficiencies, are increasingly prevalent due to a variety of environmental, dietary, and health-related factors. These issues collectively reduce the availability of essential nutrients in our food supply and hinder their absorption in the body. The key reasons for this trend include the following:

1. **Degraded Soil Quality**: Modern agricultural practices have significantly degraded soil health. The widespread use of herbicides like glyphosate disrupts the soil microbiome by killing microorganisms that play a vital role in nutrient creation and cycling. Synthetic fertilizers, while effective in replenishing nitrogen, phosphate, and potassium, fail to restore the full spectrum of nutrients needed for healthy soil. Furthermore, mono-cropping, the practice of growing the same crop repeatedly, depletes soil nutrients, whereas crop rotation can help replenish them.
2. **Processed Food Consumption**: Diets high in processed and ultra-

processed foods lack the essential vitamins and minerals necessary for good health. These foods are energy-dense but nutrient-poor, making it challenging for individuals to meet their daily nutritional needs.

3. **Chronic Disease Prevalence**: Chronic illnesses such as diabetes, cardiovascular conditions, and autoimmune disorders increase the body's need for nutrients. These conditions place additional stress on bodily systems, requiring higher levels of vitamins and minerals to support immune function, repair tissues, and regulate metabolic processes.

4. **Chemical Exposure and Pollution**: Exposure to environmental pollutants and chemicals raises oxidative stress in the body, which increases the demand for nutrients such as magnesium, zinc, and selenium that support detoxification and cellular repair processes.

5. **Increased Body Weight**: The global rise in average body weight has created additional nutritional challenges. Larger body sizes increase the demand for essential nutrients, meaning that the same dietary intake might be insufficient for individuals with higher body weights.

6. **Medications**: Certain medications, including proton pump inhibitors (PPIs), antibiotics, steroids, and oral contraceptives, interfere with nutrient absorption or actively deplete the body's nutrient stores. For instance, PPIs reduce stomach acid, which is essential for absorbing magnesium and vitamin B12.

7. **Poor Gut Health**: Gut health plays a critical role in nutrient absorption. Chronic inflammation, dysbiosis (an imbalance in gut bacteria), or conditions like irritable bowel syndrome (IBS) can impair the colon's ability to absorb nutrients efficiently. A compromised gut lining further limits the body's ability to extract nutrients from food.

8. **Increased Nutrient Requirements**: Modern lifestyles characterized by high stress levels, poor sleep, and exposure to environmental toxins increase the body's nutrient demands. Combined with declining food nutrient density, these factors have led to widespread deficiencies.

Nutrients to Support Postnatal Depletion

The postpartum period is a time of intense physical and emotional transformation. Recovering from pregnancy and childbirth, producing breast milk, and adapting to the mental load of motherhood place immense nutritional demands on the body - demands that often go unmet.

While a whole-food, nutrient-dense diet forms the foundation of recovery, individual nutrient needs can vary widely depending on your birth experience, breastfeeding status, stress levels, and overall health. That's why testing, personalization, and practitioner support are essential.

Tools like Hair Tissue Mineral Analysis (HTMA) or blood panels can help pinpoint deficiencies and imbalances, guiding a more tailored supplement and food approach (see Chapter 21 for details on HTMA testing).

Below is a summary of key nutrients commonly depleted during the first year postpartum - along with their roles in recovery and signs that your body might be lacking them.

Iron

- **Symptoms of Deficiency:** Fatigue, hair loss, dizziness, pale skin, shortness of breath, frequent infections.
- **Why It Matters:** Iron is crucial for red blood cell production, energy, immune resilience, and cognitive clarity. Blood loss during birth and breastfeeding can deplete stores rapidly.
- **Top Sources:** Grass-fed beef, liver, lentils, spinach, quinoa, pumpkin seeds.

Vitamin B12

- **Symptoms of Deficiency:** Low energy, depression, poor memory, tingling hands/feet, anemia.
- **Why It Matters:** Vital for nervous system health, mood stability, and energy metabolism. Low B12 is especially common in vegetarian or vegan

mothers.
- **Top Sources:** Animal products—eggs, dairy, meat, seafood; fortified plant-based milks.

Vitamin B6

- **Symptoms of Deficiency:** Irritability, insomnia, mood swings, PMS-like symptoms, cracked lips.
- **Why It Matters:** B6 supports neurotransmitter production (like serotonin and GABA), hormone metabolism, and adrenal health—making it a key player in mood and stress resilience postpartum.
- **Top Sources:** Bananas, chicken, turkey, sunflower seeds, sweet potatoes.

Choline

- **Symptoms of Deficiency:** Memory issues, brain fog, muscle tension.
- **Why It Matters:** Crucial for brain development (in baby) and cognitive health (in mother). Supports nerve signaling, liver function, and mental focus.
- **Top Sources:** Egg yolks, liver, beef, chicken, fish, soybeans.

Zinc

- **Symptoms of Deficiency:** Slow wound healing, skin issues, low immunity, thinning hair.
- **Why It Matters:** Supports tissue repair, immune function, skin health, and hormone balance. Zinc is often depleted during pregnancy and breastfeeding.
- **Top Sources:** Oysters, beef, pumpkin seeds, chickpeas, cashews.

Magnesium

- **Symptoms of Deficiency:** Anxiety, muscle cramps, insomnia, headaches, constipation.
- **Why It Matters:** A calming mineral that regulates stress, mood, blood sugar, and muscle function. Crucial for adrenal recovery and sleep.
- **Top Sources:** Almonds, spinach, dark chocolate, avocado, legumes.

Vitamin D

- **Symptoms of Deficiency:** Low mood, bone pain, frequent illness, fatigue.
- **Why It Matters:** Supports mood (via serotonin), immunity, bone health, and hormonal regulation. Often low in indoor-bound, breastfeeding, or winter-born mothers.
- **Top Sources:** Sunlight, oily fish, eggs, fortified foods.

Calcium

- **Symptoms of Deficiency:** Muscle twitching, brittle nails, irritability, poor sleep.
- **Why It Matters:** Needed for bone strength, muscle and nerve function, and maintaining stable moods. During breastfeeding, calcium is diverted to milk supply, pulling from maternal stores.
- **Top Sources:** Sardines, leafy greens, tahini, yogurt, aged cheese.

Iodine

- **Symptoms of Deficiency:** Fatigue, low thyroid function, dry skin, poor concentration.
- **Why It Matters:** Essential for thyroid hormone production and metabolism. Pregnancy and lactation increase iodine requirements.
- **Top Sources:** Seaweed, iodized salt, dairy, fish, eggs.

Folate (Vitamin B9)

- **Symptoms of Deficiency:** Fatigue, poor healing, irritability, brain fog.
- **Why It Matters:** Needed for tissue regeneration, red blood cell formation, and nervous system health. Use the active form (methylfolate) if you have an MTHFR gene mutation.
- **Top Sources:** Leafy greens, lentils, avocados, asparagus, beets.

Vitamin A

- **Symptoms of Deficiency:** Dry eyes or skin, poor immune response, low night vision.
- **Why It Matters:** Supports skin healing, immune resilience, and hormone balance. Also vital for thyroid function and mucous membrane health.
- **Top Sources:** Liver, egg yolks, butter, carrots, sweet potatoes (from beta-carotene).

Selenium

- **Symptoms of Deficiency:** Sluggish metabolism, frequent colds, dry skin, weak nails.
- **Why It Matters:** A key antioxidant that supports thyroid function, immune strength, and detoxification.
- **Top Sources:** Brazil nuts (1–2/day is enough), tuna, turkey, sunflower seeds.

Vitamin C

- **Symptoms of Deficiency:** Easy bruising, poor wound healing, frequent infections.
- **Why It Matters:** Essential for collagen production, iron absorption, immune function, and tissue repair—particularly after a tear or C-section.

- **Top Sources:** Bell peppers, kiwi, citrus, strawberries, broccoli.

Omega-3 Fatty Acids (DHA & EPA)

- **Symptoms of Deficiency:** Brain fog, dry skin, irritability, low mood.
- **Why It Matters:** Crucial for maternal mood, baby's brain development, and inflammation reduction. Strongly linked to postpartum depression prevention.
- **Top Sources:** Sardines, salmon, mackerel, chia seeds, flaxseed oil.

Amino Acids (from Protein)

- **Symptoms of Deficiency:** Weakness, slow healing, poor skin/hair quality, low immunity.
- **Why It Matters:** Protein supplies amino acids required for muscle repair, enzyme function, neurotransmitter production, and hormone synthesis.
- **Top Sources:** Eggs, grass-fed meats, wild-caught fish, legumes, quinoa, organic tofu.

What About Supplements?

Even with the best intentions, most mothers struggle to get everything they need through food alone - especially during the first year. In many cases, targeted supplementation based on symptoms and test results is not just helpful, but necessary.

Besides taking a high quality multi-vitamin and mineral supplement, it is a good idea to personalize your supplement intake, below is an overview of the tests that can do this.

Tests That Measure Nutrient Levels

1. Standard Blood Tests (Conventional Pathology)

Often ordered by GPs or integrative doctors to assess immediate nutrient status in blood serum or plasma.

- **Iron Studies**: Ferritin (storage), Serum Iron, Transferrin Saturation, TIBC
- **Vitamin D (25-Hydroxy D)**: Best marker for vitamin D stores
- **Vitamin B12 and Folate**: Serum levels (note: may not show functional deficiency)
- **Magnesium (Serum)**: Not very accurate—only 1% of magnesium is in the blood
- **Zinc & Copper**: Plasma or serum levels (zinc should ideally be higher than copper)
- **Calcium**: Serum calcium (though tightly regulated and not the best marker of true deficiency)
- **Phosphate**: Often tested with calcium to assess bone and metabolic status
- **Full Blood Count (FBC)**: Can show indirect signs of nutrient deficiencies (e.g., B12, folate, iron)

2. Functional Tests (More Comprehensive & Cellular)

Used by nutritionists, naturopaths, and functional medicine doctors to assess how well nutrients are being utilized, not just how much is circulating in the blood.

- **Organic Acids Test (OAT)** – *Urine-based:* Assesses functional levels of B vitamins, antioxidants, amino acids, and mitochondrial nutrients. Can identify nutrient cofactor deficiencies indirectly through metabolic markers. Commonly used to assess energy, mood, gut, and detox

function
- **Hair Tissue Mineral Analysis (HTMA)** – *Hair sample:* Shows long-term mineral status (calcium, magnesium, potassium, sodium, zinc, copper, selenium). Can also reflect **toxic metals** (mercury, lead, aluminum, etc.). Useful for spotting chronic imbalances not visible in blood
- **Micronutrient Test (e.g., SpectraCell)** – *Blood test measuring nutrient function in white blood cells:* Assesses **intracellular** levels of **vitamins, minerals, amino acids, antioxidants** over several months. More accurate for nutrients like magnesium, selenium, B6, and chromium
- **Homocysteine** – *Blood test:* Elevated levels can signal **B6, B12, or folate deficiency**, even when serum levels appear normal. Also a cardiovascular risk marker

Key Takeaway: Your Needs Are Unique

Postpartum recovery isn't one-size-fits-all. Your body might need more B6 for mood, more magnesium for sleep, or more choline for brain health - and no standard plan can fully predict that.

By listening to your body, tracking symptoms, and considering personalized testing, you can nourish yourself more effectively and restore balance more quickly.

The Broader Health Impacts of Nutritional Deficiencies

When your body is running on empty, the effects go far beyond simply feeling tired or "off." Over time, nutritional deficiencies can quietly erode your physical health, mental well-being and resilience — making it harder to show up fully as a mother and as yourself.

Your body depends on a steady supply of vitamins, minerals, and essential nutrients to function at its best. When these stores are depleted — as they often are during pregnancy, childbirth, and breastfeeding — the consequences can build over time, increasing your risk for:

- Weakened immunity, leaving you more vulnerable to frequent infections and slower healing
- Bone loss and joint issues, as deficiencies in calcium, magnesium, and vitamin D contribute to osteoporosis and joint discomfort
- Thyroid imbalances, where low levels of iodine, selenium, and zinc disrupt thyroid function and lead to fatigue, mood swings, and weight changes
- Blood sugar dysregulation, as low magnesium, chromium, fiber, and vitamin D impair insulin function and raise your risk of type 2 diabetes
- Cardiovascular strain, with low omega-3, magnesium, and potassium increasing the risk of high blood pressure and heart disease
- Autoimmune vulnerability, where nutrient imbalances contribute to chronic inflammation and reduced immune regulation
- Mental health and mood issues such as anxiety, brain fog, emotional exhaustion because nourishment isn't just about the body — it's essential for a balanced mind. When you're missing key nutrients like B vitamins, omega-3, magnesium, and zinc, it can affect brain chemistry and emotional resilience. This can leave you more prone to:

The Good News: Your Body Can Rebuild

The body is remarkably resilient. When you restore vital nutrients, you don't just feel a little better — you reclaim your energy, clarity, and strength.

- **Energy revival**: Iron, B vitamins, and magnesium help fight fatigue and restore steady, all-day vitality so you can keep up with motherhood without feeling drained
- **Emotional balance**: Omega-3, zinc, and vitamin D help regulate mood, calm the nervous system, and reduce anxiety, helping you feel more like yourself again
- **Physical recovery**: Calcium, protein, vitamin C, and other nutrients help

rebuild tissue, strengthen bones, and support healing after birth
- **Disease prevention**: A well-nourished body is better protected against long-term risks like heart disease, diabetes, and osteoporosis

Further nutritional guidance is provided in chapter 6 which outlines a 2 week nutrient dense meal plan. This meal plan also helps restore gut health and reduce chronic inflammation which are covered in the next chapters.

4

Restoring Gut Health

Gut health plays a crucial role in the postpartum period, assisting with the physical and emotional transition and recovery process. This is because the gut microbiome – a vast community of bacteria, fungi, and other microorganisms – directly impacts digestion, immunity, hormone balance, and mental well-being. Pregnancy and childbirth can significantly disrupt this delicate ecosystem, leaving many mothers vulnerable to digestive issues, inflammation, fatigue, and even mood disturbances.

During pregnancy, hormonal shifts – especially fluctuations in estrogen and progesterone – alter the gut microbiome's composition, affecting nutrient absorption, immune function, and inflammation levels. These changes can contribute to common postpartum concerns such as bloating, constipation, and food sensitivities. Additionally, gut imbalances have been linked to pregnancy complications like gestational diabetes and preeclampsia, further underscoring the importance of restoring gut health after birth.

Beyond the mother's own well-being, the postpartum gut microbiome also plays a foundational role in shaping her baby's health. Research shows that a mother's microbiome is directly passed to her child – particularly through vaginal birth and breastfeeding – helping to establish the infant's gut flora, immune function, and metabolic health. Babies born via cesarean delivery, who miss this initial exposure, often have an altered microbiome, which has been associated with an increased risk of allergies, autoimmune conditions, and metabolic disorders later in life.

How Routine Antibiotics During Birth Can Disrupt the Gut

Many mothers are unknowingly administered intravenous antibiotics during labor - often as a routine precaution in case an emergency cesarean becomes necessary during a high-risk vaginal birth (such as with twins), due to hospital policy for premature babies, or to reduce the risk of Group B Streptococcus (GBS) transmission.

While these interventions can be essential and life-saving, they can also disrupt the balance of beneficial gut bacteria. Antibiotics don't differentiate between helpful and harmful microbes, so they may inadvertently wipe out protective strains, leaving room for opportunistic pathogens to thrive. This disruption can affect digestion, immune function, mental health, and energy levels in the postpartum period. For breastfeeding mothers, it may also impact the infant's developing microbiome, as microbial diversity passed through breast milk might be reduced. If you received antibiotics during labor or a cesarean, it's especially important to gently support your microbiome with fermented foods, fiber, and rest – and to allow your body the time it needs to recover from this invisible internal shift.

Common signs that may be linked to IV antibiotic-related dysbiosis include:

- Persistent bloating or sugar cravings postpartum
- Recurrent thrush (in mum or baby)
- Food intolerances that weren't present before
- Vaginal or digestive yeast overgrowth
- Low mood or anxious feelings with no clear emotional trigger

For postpartum mothers, restoring gut health is a critical step toward recovery and long-term vitality. Nourishing the microbiome through a balanced diet, probiotic-rich foods and mindful lifestyle choices can support digestion, reduce inflammation, balance hormones, and enhance overall energy levels. A healthy gut can also improve mood stability, as the gut-brain axis plays a major role in regulating neurotransmitters like serotonin – key to emotional well-being in the postpartum period.

Interestingly, while men and women share a similar gut microbiome structure, women experience more fluctuations due to hormonal cycles, pregnancy, and menopause. This makes postpartum recovery a particularly vulnerable time for gut imbalances, as these imbalances can magnify conditions like postpartum thyroid dysfunction, autoimmune flares, and metabolic challenges. Additionally, gut dysbiosis has been linked to conditions like PCOS (polycystic ovary syndrome), which affects an estimated 10% of women globally. Women with PCOS often experience insulin resistance, irregular menstrual cycles, and metabolic dysfunction – issues deeply connected to gut health. By prioritizing gut restoration in the postpartum phase, mothers not only support their own recovery but also set the stage for hormonal balance and overall wellness in the years to come.

Common Signs of Poor Gut Health

- **Digestive issues:** Persistent bloating, diarrhea, or constipation may signal gut microbiota imbalances that disrupt digestion.
- **Chronic fatigue:** Poor gut health can limit nutrient absorption, resulting in reduced energy and long-term fatigue.
- **Food intolerance:** Imbalances in gut bacteria can impair the breakdown of specific foods, causing discomfort or inflammation.
- **Frequent illnesses:** A weakened microbiome compromises immune function, leaving the body vulnerable to infections.
- **Skin conditions:** Gut dysbiosis can influence skin health through the gut-skin axis, leading to acne, eczema, or other conditions.
- **Unexplained weight changes:** Disruptions in the gut microbiome can alter metabolic pathways, affecting weight regulation.
- **Brain fog or poor concentration:** Dysbiosis may impair cognitive

function due to the bidirectional gut-brain axis.
- **Sleep disturbances:** Microbiota imbalances can affect melatonin production, leading to poor sleep quality or insomnia.
- **Sugar cravings:** Certain gut bacteria thrive on sugar and may influence cravings to support their growth.
- **Bad breath:** Gut issues can lead to a buildup of volatile sulfur compounds and other waste gases from dysbiosis, poor digestion, or sluggish detoxification, all of which contribute to halitosis.
- **Mood disorders:** Gut dysbiosis may reduce serotonin synthesis, exacerbating anxiety or depression.
- **Joint pain or inflammation:** Imbalanced gut bacteria can increase systemic inflammation, contributing to conditions like arthritis.
- **Irritable bowel syndrome (IBS) symptoms:** Gut imbalances often underlie IBS, causing abdominal pain and irregular bowel habits.
- **Allergies or sensitivities:** A disrupted gut lining may allow allergens to enter the bloodstream, triggering immune responses.
- **Slow metabolism or low energy levels:** A poor microbiome can impair energy metabolism, leading to sluggishness and weight gain.

Phase 1: Gentle Gut Restoration

If you've just had a baby and feel overwhelmed or unsure where to start, this phase is about making small, nourishing changes that add up – without stress or restriction. Healing your gut if you are breastfeeding requires a gentle, supportive approach rather than intense detoxification. Your body is already working hard to nourish both you and your baby, and any drastic gut healing protocol – such as extreme elimination diets, aggressive detox supplements, or fasting – could release toxins too quickly, potentially affecting breast milk and your energy levels. Instead of focusing on rapid detox, the goal in this phase is to reduce inflammation, remove common gut irritants, and lay a strong foundation for long-term healing without overwhelming your body.

By prioritizing nutrient-dense, gut-supportive foods, hydration, and digestion-friendly habits, you can start to restore balance in your microbiome while ensuring that your milk supply and energy remain strong. This phase is about nourishing and rebuilding – not depriving or overburdening your system.

Step 1: Remove Common Gut Irritants

A well-functioning gut thrives when it's not constantly exposed to inflammatory foods or substances that disrupt the microbiome. However, it's important to avoid over-restriction, as cutting out too many foods can increase stress and make it harder to get the nutrients you and your baby need. These are the top gut irritants to avoid:

- **Ultra-processed foods:** Packaged snacks, refined sugars, seed oils, and preservatives can contribute to gut dysbiosis and inflammation.
- **Excess caffeine and alcohol:** Both can stress digestion, impact gut lining integrity, and affect your baby's sleep through breastmilk.
- **Artificial sweeteners & gums:** These can disrupt beneficial bacteria and contribute to bloating or gas.
- **Common inflammatory foods (if sensitive):** Some people—especially those with gut issues—react to foods like gluten, dairy, and soy with symptoms such as bloating, skin flare-ups (like eczema), or discomfort. If you or your baby experience these symptoms (especially during breastfeeding), reducing these foods may help calm inflammation and improve digestion.

Step 2: Prioritize Nutrient-Dense, Gut-Healing Foods

Instead of focusing on what to remove, the most sustainable way to heal your gut is by adding in foods that nourish and restore.

Gut-Healing Super Foods:

- **Bone broth:** Rich in collagen, amino acids, and minerals to support gut

lining repair.
- **Fermented foods** (start with small amounts initially to avoid digestive discomfort): Kefir, sauerkraut, coconut yogurt, miso, and kimchi help repopulate good bacteria.
- **Healthy fats:** Avocado, extra virgin olive oil, grass-fed butter/ghee, and omega-3-rich fish lower inflammation and support brain health.
- **Prebiotic fiber:** Cooked and cooled potatoes/rice (resistant starch), onions, garlic, leeks, asparagus, and green bananas feed good bacteria.
- **Easily digestible proteins:** Slow-cooked meats, pastured eggs, wild-caught fish, and collagen peptides support recovery.
- **Eat the rainbow:** Include a wide variety of fresh fruits, vegetables, herbs, and spices in your diet.

Step 3: Support Digestion & Nutrient Absorption

Even the most nourishing foods won't be effective if your body can't digest and absorb them properly. A sluggish digestive system is often common in postpartum women and can result in bloating, constipation, nutrient deficiencies, and discomfort.

Simple Ways to Improve Digestion:

- **Chew food thoroughly:** Digestion begins in the mouth. Slow, mindful eating helps reduce bloating and improves absorption.
- **Eat in a relaxed state:** Stress shifts the body into "fight or flight," reducing digestive enzyme production. Try deep breathing before meals and being in the present moment when eating.
- **Incorporate digestive support:** Herbal teas like ginger, fennel, and chamomile can soothe the gut. Apple cider vinegar or digestive bitters before meals are also helpful.

Step 4: Prioritize Hydration & Electrolytes

Breastfeeding significantly increases fluid needs, and dehydration can slow digestion and contribute to fatigue, constipation, and headaches.
Best Ways to Stay Hydrated:

- **Filtered water:** Aim for at least 2.5–3L per day, especially if breastfeeding.
- **Coconut water:** A natural source of electrolytes to replenish minerals.
- **Lemon water with sea salt:** Supports hydration and gentle detoxification.
- **Herbal teas:** Chamomile, peppermint, and rooibos can be soothing.

Establishing Foundational Steps for Gut Health

By following these gentle, foundational steps, you're giving your gut the space it needs to heal without shocking your system or compromising your milk supply. This phase sets the groundwork for deeper microbiome restoration and hormonal balance in later stages, ensuring that both you and your baby thrive.

Phase 2: Deeper Microbiome Restoration

Once your body has had time to adjust and regain strength, the next section of this book will take things further – focusing on microbiome diversity, gut lining repair and long-term digestive resilience. If you're experiencing persistent bloating, food sensitivities, brain fog, or low energy, this phase will offer a structured protocol to fully restore your gut microbiome and rebuild your resilience.

5

Eating to Fight Chronic Inflammation

Why an Anti-Inflammatory Diet Matters After Birth

During the fourth trimester—and well into the first year—your body is working hard to repair tissues, regulate shifting hormones, recover from nutrient loss, and keep up with the physical and emotional demands of caring for a newborn. While this period is often seen as natural and expected, it's also a time when inflammation can quietly delay recovery, drain energy and affect mental clarity and mood.

In this context, an anti-inflammatory diet isn't just about long-term disease prevention—it's a practical and powerful tool to support healing, energy, hormone balance, and mental well-being during this critical time of repair and rebuilding.

An anti-inflammatory diet has gained increasing attention in both scientific research and wellness circles for its ability to improve energy levels, support overall health, and reduce the risk of chronic disease. It emphasizes foods that reduce oxidative stress, calm the immune system, and promote healing—such as colorful fruits and vegetables, omega-3-rich fish, nuts, seeds and antioxidant-rich herbs and spices.

Chronic inflammation, unlike the short-term immune response that occurs during injury or infection, can persist silently over time. It is now widely recognized as a contributing factor in the development of numerous health conditions, including heart disease, type 2 diabetes, autoimmune disorders, neurodegenerative diseases, and certain cancers. It can be triggered by poor diet, environmental toxins, ongoing stress, sleep deprivation, and other lifestyle factors—many of which are common in early motherhood.

With an estimated 60% of adults worldwide living with at least one inflammation-related chronic illness, prioritizing nutrition and lifestyle choices that lower inflammation is essential—not just for long-term prevention, but for feeling better now.

Subtle signs of chronic inflammation that may be affecting you:

- **Fatigue and low energy**: Feeling constantly drained despite rest
- **Joint pain and muscle aches**: Ongoing discomfort without a clear cause
- **Digestive issues**: Bloating, gut discomfort, or IBS-like symptoms
- **Brain fog and memory lapses**: Trouble concentrating or feeling mentally "off"
- **Skin conditions**: Acne, eczema, or unexplained rashes
- **Frequent infections**: Weakened immunity or slow wound healing
- **Unexplained weight changes**: Disrupted metabolism or appetite shifts

Whether you're navigating the early stages of postpartum or looking to rebuild your vitality well into your second year of motherhood, adopting an anti-inflammatory approach to eating can be a gentle yet powerful way to support your body's natural healing processes.

How an Anti-Inflammatory Diet Supports Postpartum Recovery

- **Energy & Hormonal Balance:** Postpartum fatigue is common, and inflammation can further drain energy levels and disrupt hormonal balance. An anti-inflammatory diet rich in omega-3, antioxidants, and whole foods helps stabilize blood sugar, reduce brain fog, and support adrenal function, improving overall vitality. Avoiding inflammatory foods like refined sugars and processed oils can enhance mood and prevent energy crashes.
- **Healing & Tissue Repair:** After childbirth, the body undergoes a natural healing process, which can be slowed by chronic inflammation. Nutrient-dense foods such as leafy greens, berries, wild-caught fish, and healthy fats provide essential compounds that aid in tissue repair, reduce swelling, and promote faster recovery from delivery or C-section scars.
- **Reducing Risk of Postpartum Depression & Anxiety:** Inflammation has been linked to mental health challenges, including postpartum depression. A diet high in anti-inflammatory foods, such as turmeric, fatty fish, and fermented foods, can help regulate neurotransmitters and gut health, both of which play a key role in mood stabilization and stress resilience.

Inflammatory Foods to Avoid

If you're dealing with chronic inflammation and its ongoing symptoms, it may be worth eliminating certain foods for a few months to help reset your body. Individuals with suboptimal gut health often struggle to digest these foods, which can contribute to persistent inflammation and discomfort.

Conventional Dairy Products

Dairy can be a source of inflammation, particularly for those with lactose intolerance or sensitivity to dairy proteins like casein. Conventional dairy, often produced with hormones and antibiotics, can exacerbate inflammatory reactions and contribute to digestive issues, joint pain, and skin inflammation. Studies suggest that dairy consumption may increase biomarkers of inflammation, particularly among people with existing sensitivities.

Wheat and Gluten Containing Grains

While gluten-containing grains are a staple in many diets, their inflammatory effects are particularly concerning for those with gluten sensitivities or celiac disease. Even in those without diagnosed sensitivities, gluten is believed to promote inflammation in some individuals by increasing intestinal permeability, commonly referred to as "leaky gut". This condition has been linked to various autoimmune and inflammatory diseases.

The gluten protein is found in wheat, barley, rye, spelt and their derivatives. For individuals sensitive to gluten, eliminating it may reduce chronic inflammation, irritation of the digestive tract and improve overall well-being. Some studies suggest that reducing inflammation through dietary changes, including the removal of gluten, may support better mental health outcomes, potentially alleviating symptoms of anxiety.

In sensitive individuals, consuming gluten can lead to digestive discomfort, fatigue, and inflammation throughout the body, including the brain. Research suggests that inflammation may play a role in the development or exacerbation of anxiety symptoms in some people.

By opting for gluten-free alternatives, individuals can potentially improve their overall well-being and manage anxiety symptoms more effectively. Here are some gluten-free options that can be incorporated into a balanced diet:

Gluten-Free Options:

- **Quinoa:** Protein and fiber-rich gluten-free grain.
- **Rice:** Brown, white, or wild varieties.
- **Corn:** Cornmeal, polenta, and tortillas.
- **Gluten-free oats:** Ensure they are labeled to avoid cross-contamination.

- **Legumes:** Beans, lentils, and chickpeas are gluten-free and fiber-rich.

Sugar

Added sugar, especially in high amounts, can lead to chronic inflammation by stimulating pro-inflammatory cytokines. Frequent sugar consumption has been associated with insulin resistance, obesity, and increased risk of type 2 diabetes – all of which have inflammatory components. Studies indicate that a diet high in refined sugar may elevate C-reactive protein (CRP) levels, a key marker of inflammation.

High sugar intake also has a negative effect on the gut microbiome, leading to an imbalance of beneficial bacteria and promoting the growth of harmful microbes. Reducing sugar can help restore this balance, which not only reduces inflammation but supports better digestion, immunity, and overall health.

Refined Seed Oils

Refined seed oils have become a staple in the modern food industry due to their low cost, mild flavor, and high smoke point. They are widely used in processed foods, restaurant cooking, and home kitchens. However, their widespread use has significant health implications, and most people are unknowingly consuming them in excess.

While deep-fried and packaged foods are the most obvious sources of vegetable oils, they are also hidden in baby formula, plant-based milks, salad dressings, sauces, and baked goods. As their consumption has increased, so have concerns about their impact on inflammation, oxidative stress, and chronic disease risk.

Canola oil is one of the most widely consumed vegetable oils today, with its production having tripled in just a few decades. In 2022 alone, the U.S. produced 2.9 million metric tons of canola oil. Similarly, soybean and sunflower oils dominate processed foods, further increasing overall omega-6 consumption.

Why refined seed oils are problematic:

1. **High in Omega-6 Fatty Acids, Leading to Inflammation:** Seed oils like soybean, sunflower, and canola oil are high in omega-6 polyunsaturated fatty acids (PUFAs). While omega-6 is essential in small amounts, excessive consumption disrupts the balance of omega-6 to omega-3 fatty acids. This imbalance contributes to chronic low-grade inflammation, a key driver of heart disease, arthritis, diabetes, and other inflammatory conditions.
2. **Oxidative Stress and Cellular Damage:** The industrial processing of these oils involves high heat and chemical refining, creating harmful byproducts like aldehydes and oxidized lipids. These compounds contribute to oxidative stress, which accelerates cellular aging and is linked to cancer, neurodegenerative diseases, and metabolic disorders.
3. **Increased Risk of Cardiovascular Disease:** Some research suggests that diets high in omega-6 seed oils may disrupt cholesterol balance and promote systemic inflammation, increasing the risk of heart disease. Although omega-6 fats play a role in the body, excessive intake, especially in the absence of anti-inflammatory omega-3, can be harmful to cardiovascular health.
4. **Toxic Byproducts from High-Heat Processing:** Refined seed oils undergo deodorizing, bleaching, and degumming, all of which expose the oils to extremely high temperatures. These processes not only strip away beneficial nutrients but also create harmful trans fats and toxic oxidation products that further contribute to inflammation and metabolic dysfunction.
5. **Genetically Modified Crops and Chemical Residues:** The majority of seed oil crops, such as soy, canola, and safflower, are genetically modified (GM) to tolerate repeated applications of herbicides and pesticides, particularly glyphosate. According to the U.S. Food and Drug Administration (FDA), around 95% of canola and 94% of soybean crops are genetically engineered to survive heavy chemical exposure. Residues from these chemicals have been linked to hormone disruption,

gut health disturbances, and potential cancer risks.

Healthier Alternatives

To reduce inflammation and oxidative stress, opt for minimally processed, nutrient-dense fats that support overall health, such as:

- **Extra Virgin Olive Oil:** Rich in antioxidants and monounsaturated fats, supports heart health
- **Coconut Oil:** Provides stable saturated fats, ideal for high-heat cooking
- **Ghee:** Packed with fat-soluble vitamins and beneficial short-chain fatty acids
- **Avocado Oil:** High in monounsaturated fats, resistant to oxidation

Switching from refined seed oils to these healthier options can protect against inflammation, support optimal metabolic function, and promote long-term wellness.

6

Postnatal Meal Plan - 2 Weeks

As a busy mother of three I know how overwhelming it can feel when you're juggling everything, and now, on top of that, you've been handed a ton of information about nourishing yourself. That's exactly why I've created a simple, practical meal plan to take the guesswork out of healthy eating with real life in mind. It helps you cook once and enjoy leftovers for lunch, reuse ingredients throughout the week to save time and money, and ensure every meal is nutrient-dense, delicious, and easy to prepare.

You spend so much energy caring for everyone else, but you deserve to feel nourished, energized, and supported too. This meal plan was created to bring balance, vitality, and ease into your life, without adding more to your plate.

This isn't about dieting or quick fixes. It's about real food that truly fuels both your body and soul. Thoughtfully designed to support you beyond postpartum recovery and restore your health, this meal plan will:

- **Nourish hormones** with key hormone-supporting foods such as cruciferous vegetables, flaxseeds, healthy fats, fiber, polyphenols, and micronutrients that help balance estrogen, progesterone, and cortisol.
- **Support gut health** with a diverse range of plants, fiber, polyphenols and probiotic-rich foods like kefir and sauerkraut.

- **Provide ample protein** to aid in postpartum recovery, tissue repair, and sustained energy.
- **Replenish essential nutrients** like zinc, iron, and choline to support healing and vitality.
- **Lower inflammation** by incorporating anti-inflammatory ingredients and avoiding common gut irritants.
- **Be easy and delicious**, with minimal preparation and meals that make the most of leftovers.
- **Minimize food waste** by using ingredients multiple times throughout the week—staples like roast chicken, sweet potatoes, quinoa, and greens appear in several meals.
- **Remove the stress of counting calories**, focusing instead on feeling nourished and eating until you are satisfied.
- **Promote blood sugar balance** with low sugar meals that are high in protein and complex carbohydrates for steady energy levels and a stable mood throughout the day.

Week 1

Day 1

- **Breakfast:** Smoothie with kefir or Greek yogurt, spinach, frozen berries, ½ banana, chia seeds, 1 date, a scoop of collagen powder, flaxseeds, ice and water.
- **Snack:** Carrot sticks with hummus and a handful of almonds.
- **Lunch:** Chicken salad with mixed greens, avocado, cherry tomatoes, cucumber, pumpkin seeds - buy a hot roast chicken from the shop.
- **Dinner:** Oven baked salmon with olive oil, garlic, and lemon, served with steamed broccoli, roasted sweet potatoes, and quinoa.

Day 2

- **Breakfast:** Avocado toast on gluten-free sourdough with 2 fried eggs, fresh herbs, and a sprinkle of sesame seeds.
- **Snack:** Coconut yogurt with hemp seeds, walnuts, cacao nibs and a fruit of your choice.
- **Lunch:** Leftover salmon and quinoa on a bed of greens with tahini dressing and a side of fermented sauerkraut.
- **Dinner:** Beef stir-fry with bell peppers, carrots, snap peas, and ginger over cauliflower rice.

Day 3

- **Breakfast:** Chia pudding made with coconut milk, flaxseeds, cinnamon, and fresh blueberries.
- **Snack:** Handful of mixed nuts and a few dark chocolate squares.
- **Lunch:** Turkey lettuce wraps with shredded carrots, cucumber, avocado, and a squeeze of lime and organic mayonnaise.
- **Dinner:** Coconut curry chicken with zucchini, spinach, bell peppers, and wild rice.

Day 4

- **Breakfast:** Scrambled eggs with spinach and smoked salmon, served with gluten-free or traditional sourdough toast and avocado.
- **Snack:** Kefir smoothie with frozen berries, a handful of spinach, chia seeds, ice and water.
- **Lunch:** Leftover coconut curry chicken over greens with pumpkin seeds.
- **Dinner:** Baked cod with roasted Brussels sprouts, mashed sweet potatoes, and sautéed kale.

Day 5

- **Breakfast:** Oatmeal with coconut milk, berries, almond butter, flaxseeds, and cinnamon.

- **Snack:** Sliced apple with almond butter and a sprinkle of pumpkin seeds.
- **Lunch:** Roasted veggie salad with boiled eggs, avocado, mixed beans, and tahini dressing.
- **Dinner:** Lamb meatballs with zucchini noodles, marinara sauce, and a side of sauerkraut.

Day 6

- **Breakfast:** Smoothie with coconut yogurt, spinach, hemp seeds, mixed berries, banana, water and ice.
- **Snack:** Coconut water, walnuts and fruit of your choice
- **Lunch:** Leftover lamb meatballs with roasted veggies and greens.
- **Dinner:** Roast chicken thighs with rosemary, roasted carrots, parsnips, and steamed asparagus.

Day 7

- **Breakfast:** Poached eggs over gluten-free or traditional sourdough toast with sautéed mushrooms and tomatoes.
- **Snack:** Celery sticks with almond butter.
- **Lunch:** Salad with leftover roast chicken, mixed greens, olives, cucumber, and an olive oil dressing.
- **Dinner:** Wild-caught shrimp stir-fry with bell peppers, onions, snap peas, and quinoa.

Week 2

Day 1

- **Breakfast:** Smoothie with banana, spinach, frozen berries, 1 date, chia seeds, protein powder, kefir, ice and water.

- **Snack:** Mixed nuts, seeds, and dark chocolate.
- **Lunch:** Turkey and avocado lettuce wrap with sauerkraut.
- **Dinner:** Grass-fed beef stew with carrots, potatoes, onions, and celery.

Day 2

- **Breakfast:** Chia pudding with coconut milk, berries and hemp seeds.
- **Snacks:** Apple with almonds and dark chocolate.
- **Lunch:** Leftover beef stew with a side of greens.
- **Dinner:** Roasted salmon with lemon and chives, Brussels sprouts, and mashed sweet potatoes.

Day 3

- **Breakfast:** Scrambled eggs with sautéed kale and cherry tomatoes.
- **Snacks:** Coconut yogurt with pumpkin seeds and a cup of bone broth.
- **Lunch:** Quinoa salad with roasted veggies, chickpeas, avocado, and sauerkraut.
- **Dinner:** Herb-crusted lamb chops with roasted carrots and parsnips.

Day 4

- **Breakfast:** Kefir smoothie with spinach, frozen berries, flaxseeds, and protein powder.
- **Snack:** Carrot sticks with hummus.
- **Lunch:** Leftover lamb with a side salad of greens and pumpkin seeds.
- **Dinner:** Baked cod with steamed asparagus, snow peas, and wild garlic and herb rice.

Day 5

- **Breakfast:** Overnight oats with coconut milk, chia seeds, cinnamon, and banana slices.

- **Snacks:** Banana with nut butter and dark chocolate.
- **Lunch:** Tuna salad with mixed greens, olives, cucumber, and a lemon-tahini dressing.
- **Dinner:** Bone broth miso soup with rice noodles, poached eggs, bok choy, carrots, and chicken.

Day 6

- **Breakfast:** Smoothie with coconut yogurt, kefir, spinach, hemp seeds, mixed berries, and banana.
- **Snack:** Walnuts, dark chocolate and a cup of bone broth.
- **Lunch:** Chicken wrap with avocado, sauerkraut, arugula, tomato and hard-aged cheese.
- **Dinner:** Roasted beef with roasted potatoes, steamed broccoli and carrots.

Day 7

- **Breakfast:** Poached eggs on a bed of sautéed spinach and mushrooms with gluten-free toast.
- **Snack:** Coconut water and an apple.
- **Lunch:** Salad with leftover roast beef, greens, avocado, olives, and balsamic dressing.
- **Dinner:** Grilled prawns with mixed vegetable stir-fry and quinoa.
- **Evening treat:** Dark chocolate and chamomile tea.

Meal Plan Tips

- Start your meal plan the day you buy the hot chicken, or if you have the inclination, you could roast one yourself of course.
- This meal plan is designed to save you time and effort by incorporating

leftovers—especially proteins and carbohydrates—from the previous day. Be sure to check the next day's meals in advance so you can prepare enough food to carry over.

- Check your pantry: Before shopping, check what you already have to avoid duplicate purchases, especially for grains, nuts, seeds, and canned goods.
- Adjust quantities: Depending on family size and preferences, you might need to adjust the quantities of fresh produce, proteins, and grains.
- With gluten free breads there can be a lot of variation, it is worthwhile finding the most natural one available. Or if you really cannot bare to part with gluten, buy organic traditionally fermented sourdough. The fermentation breaks down gluten proteins so that they are easier to digest, thereby causing less issues for most people.
- Spices and herbs: Make sure you have a good selection of spices and herbs on hand for seasoning your meals, such as garlic powder, onion powder, cumin, paprika, and black pepper. Fresh or dried herbs and spices can enhance flavor without extra sodium or unhealthy fats. They are also high in phytonutrients.
- Sauerkraut must be bought from refrigerated section - this is the only one with probiotics.
- Choose sustainably caught wild tuna or substitute for sardines, anchovies or wild caught tinned salmon.
- Use olive oil or grass-fed butter for cooking.
- Cook enough quinoa or rice to eat the next day.
- Adequate hydration is crucial for overall health and can support breast-feeding. Aim for 8 glasses of filtered water daily, plus herbal teas (particularly chamomile, dandelion and green tea) or broths, coconut water and high-quality electrolytes if necessary.
- Use fresh and frozen produce: A variety of fruits and vegetables, whether fresh or frozen, ensures nutrient diversity and convenience.

7

The Mental and Emotional Load of Motherhood

The early years of motherhood are among the most rewarding - and demanding - seasons in a woman's life. During this time, mothers often carry not only the visible responsibilities of caring for their baby, but also an invisible weight: the mental and emotional load of parenthood.

The Mental Load

The mental load refers to the constant, behind-the-scenes thinking, planning, and organizing that keeps family life running. For mothers, this can mean remembering doctor's appointments, managing household schedules, anticipating their child's developmental needs, preparing meals, and coordinating daily routines. It's the ongoing mental checklist that never seems to end.

This invisible labor is often underestimated by others - and even by mothers themselves - but it can be a significant source of mental fatigue. Studies show that mothers, especially in the early years, are more likely to bear this planning and organizing burden, which can quietly erode their energy and emotional resilience over time.

The Emotional Load

Alongside the mental load is the emotional work of motherhood: the effort of nurturing, comforting, and regulating not only a child's emotions but also one's own. Mothers are often the emotional anchor of the family, expected to stay patient, present, and attuned to their child's needs - even when they are exhausted, overwhelmed, or uncertain themselves.

This emotional labor can be intensified by societal expectations of what a "good mother" should look like: always calm, endlessly giving, perfectly balanced. When mothers inevitably fall short of these impossible standards (because they are human), guilt and self-doubt can creep in, adding yet another layer to the emotional load.

Why the First Years Are Especially Intense

In the first years of motherhood, the mental and emotional load can feel especially heavy because so much is new - and the stakes feel so high. A mother is not only learning to care for a baby, but also adjusting to a transformed identity, shifting relationships, and a new daily reality that may include sleep deprivation, hormonal changes, and physical recovery from birth.

The constancy of early parenting - the round-the-clock feeds, the unpredictable sleep patterns, the need to be on alert at all times - means that mental rest is hard to come by. Even when a mother gets a break, it can be hard to truly switch off the planning, worrying, or troubleshooting that happens in her mind.

The Cost of an Unshared Load

When the mental and emotional load falls mostly on one person, it can lead to burnout, resentment, and a sense of isolation. It can rob mothers of joy in this precious season and make it harder to bond with their child in a relaxed, present way. That's why it's so important to name the mental and emotional load - so that mothers can seek help, share the load, and give themselves permission to rest.

Strategies & Tips

Here are 23 practical tips to help mothers cope with the mental and emotional load of motherhood, especially during those early, demanding years:

1. **Share Household Responsibilities:** Get your partner or a family member to be in charge of dividing tasks like childcare and housework. Sharing the load reduces stress by up to 30% and strengthens relationships.
2. **Let Go of Perfection:** Aim for "good enough" days instead of perfection. Every parent's journey is unique, so avoid comparing yourself to others.
3. **Take Mini Self-Care Breaks:** Even five minutes to enjoy tea, breathe, or stretch can recharge you. Small moments add up.
4. **Ask for Help:** Let family, friends, or hired help support you when they can. You don't have to do it all alone.
5. **Learn to Say 'No':** Protect your energy by saying no to commitments that feel overwhelming or unnecessary.
6. **Build Your Village:** Connect with other moms or join parenting groups in person or online. Sharing experiences makes the load lighter.
7. **Be Present in the Moment:** Practice mindfulness during everyday activities. It helps reduce stress and adds joy to small moments.
8. **Prioritize Sleep:** Sleep when you can. Use white noise, nap when your child naps, and accept nighttime help when offered.
9. **Plan Simple Routines:** Prep meals in advance, create easy schedules, and stick to simple routines to save time and energy.
10. **Move Your Body Daily:** Fit in exercise like a walk, yoga, or light stretching. It boosts mood and energy levels.
11. **Get Outside in Nature:** Spend time outdoors every day. Fresh air, sunlight, and connecting with nature can reduce stress and lift your mood.
12. **Write It Out:** Keep a journal to jot down thoughts, feelings, or goals. It's a great way to clear your mind.
13. **Stay Organized:** Use a calendar or to-do list to keep track of tasks but be flexible if plans change.

14. **Eat for Energy:** Choose whole foods like fruits, veggies, and proteins. Keep meals simple and nourishing to stay fueled.
15. **Schedule 'Me Time':** Plan regular breaks for yourself - whether it's reading, meeting a friend, or a solo coffee outing.
16. **Create Child Routines:** Set predictable routines for meals and bedtime. They help your kids feel secure and make your day smoother.
17. **Delegate Tasks:** Give specific chores to your partner or family. Sharing responsibilities lightens your mental load.
18. **Relax Your Body and Mind:** Use quick relaxation techniques like deep breathing or short meditations when you're feeling overwhelmed.
19. **Celebrate Imperfections:** Celebrate small wins and remind yourself that your best effort is enough. No one's perfect!
20. **Talk to a Therapist:** Counseling can help you process emotions, develop coping skills, and feel more supported.
21. **Focus on Gratitude:** Write down or think about small things you're grateful for each day. It can improve your mindset.
22. **Reconnect with Yourself:** Spend time on a hobby or interest outside of parenting to remind yourself of who you are beyond "mom."
23. **Remind yourself that this is just a season:** Soon enough you will look back and wonder where the time went and how your baby grew up so fast.

8

Navigating New Anxieties in Motherhood

Motherhood is a journey of deep love - but it can also bring significant emotional challenges, including anxiety. The intense demands of caring for a child, balancing work, managing the household and maintaining personal identity can create chronic stress. Add in hormonal shifts, sleep deprivation, being nutritionally depleted and the constant "mental load," and it's no surprise that many mothers find themselves overwhelmed.

Anxiety in mothers is common, yet often misunderstood or minimized. In fact, women are nearly twice as likely as men to experience an anxiety disorder at some point in their lives. According to the U.S. National Institute of Mental Health, approximately 23% of adult women experience an anxiety disorder each year - a figure that may be even higher during the childbearing and child-rearing years.

Globally, stress levels are rising. A 2021 Gallup report found that 44% of adults across 110 countries experience daily stress - but mothers, especially those balancing paid work and caregiving, face even higher pressures. A survey by *Bright Horizons* revealed that 68% of working mothers report feeling burnt out, and 52% struggle with the ongoing tension of trying to meet both work and family demands.

The Cycle of Maternal Anxiety

Anxiety is more than just occasional worry or nervousness. For mothers, it can show up as:

- **Sleep disturbances** (even beyond what comes with caring for a baby)
- **Difficulty concentrating or decision fatigue**
- **Increased irritability or mood swings**
- **Appetite changes**
- **Constant overthinking or fear of "failing" as a parent**

These challenges are often compounded by the societal pressure to "do it all" and appear to be coping effortlessly, whilst 'bouncing back' quickly. The stigma surrounding maternal mental health means many mothers don't seek help, leaving them feeling isolated and unsupported.

How Nutrition Can Support Anxiety Management

Anxiety has many contributing factors - hormonal changes, life circumstances, genetics - but evidence increasingly shows that nutrition and gut health play an important role in mental well-being. While therapy, medication, and social support can be key parts of anxiety treatment, dietary strategies can provide meaningful additional support according to research.

A landmark *randomized controlled trial* (SMILES trial, Australia) found that people following a Mediterranean-style diet for 12 weeks had a 32% greater reduction in depression symptoms compared to a control group. Similar dietary patterns benefit anxiety by supporting gut health, lowering inflammation, and improving neurotransmitter function.

Key Dietary Recommendations for Mothers

Reduce inflammatory foods

Chronic inflammation doesn't just affect your physical health - it can also play a significant role in your mental and emotional well-being. Emerging research shows a strong link between inflammation in the body and symptoms of anxiety and depression. Inflammatory chemicals called *cytokines* can interfere with neurotransmitter function in the brain, particularly serotonin and dopamine - both of which are essential for regulating mood, motivation, and emotional balance.

One of the most powerful ways to reduce chronic inflammation is through your daily food choices. Chronic inflammation can be fueled by diets high in:

- Refined sugar
- Processed carbohydrates
- Low-quality vegetable oils (like canola, soybean, and sunflower oils)
- Ultra-processed foods

These foods often disrupt the gut microbiome, damage the gut lining, and trigger an immune response that can send stress signals to the brain.

On the other hand, a nourishing, anti-inflammatory diet can help calm the nervous system, support healthy gut bacteria, and reduce systemic inflammation - creating a more stable foundation for mental health. By limiting inflammatory foods, you're not just supporting your physical vitality - you're also protecting your mental clarity, emotional resilience, and overall sense of calm.

Prioritize nutrient-dense, whole foods consisting of

- A **colorful variety of vegetables and fruits** for antioxidants and fiber
- **High-quality proteins**: grass-fed meats, pasture-raised eggs, wild-caught fish
- **Probiotic-rich foods**: sauerkraut, kefir, miso, coconut yogurt. A diverse

gut microbiome positively influences the gut-brain axis.
- **Fresh herbs and spices**: such as parsley, turmeric, ginger, garlic and cinnamon

Essential Nutrients for Reducing Anxiety

It's important to test your vitamin and mineral levels before starting supplements.

- **Magnesium**: Helps regulate the stress response and cortisol production; deficiencies are common in mothers due to increased demand.
- **Omega-3 fatty acids**: Reduce brain inflammation and support emotional resilience; found in oily fish (salmon, sardines), flaxseeds, chia.
- **Vitamin B6**: Essential for producing serotonin and GABA; found in poultry, bananas, chickpeas.
- **Zinc**: Key for neurotransmitter activity; low levels are linked to anxiety and depression. Rich sources: oysters, pumpkin seeds, beef.
- **Vitamin D**: Low levels are associated with mood disorders; safe sun exposure and fatty fish help maintain levels.
- **Iron**: Deficiency can lead to fatigue, low mood, and brain fog. Sources: liver, red meat, lentils, spinach.
- **Tryptophan**: A precursor to serotonin; found in turkey, eggs, dairy, and nuts.

The Gut-Brain Connection and Anxiety

The intricate relationship between gut health and mental well-being, known as the gut-brain axis, plays a pivotal role in managing anxiety. Emerging research highlights the potential of probiotics to improve mood. A meta-analysis found that probiotics significantly reduced symptoms of depression compared to placebo groups. Beneficial strains, such as Bifidobacterium and Lactobacillus, promote the production of serotonin and other neurotransmitters linked to mental health.

The gut microbiota – a diverse community of microorganisms in the intestines – produces neurotransmitters like serotonin, dopamine, and GABA, essential for mood regulation. Imbalances in gut microbiota, or dysbiosis, can impair neurotransmitter production and contribute to anxiety and depression.

Including probiotic-rich foods, such as yogurt, kefir, sauerkraut, and kimchi, can help restore gut balance and reduce anxiety symptoms. In addition, probiotic supplements may offer targeted support for individuals with specific gut health concerns.

Probiotics have been increasingly researched for their potential benefits in reducing anxiety, as they may help balance gut microbiota, which has a direct connection with the brain, known as the "gut-brain axis." Some of the most researched probiotics for anxiety include:

1. **Lactobacillus rhamnosus (JB-1):** Studies have shown that Lactobacillus rhamnosus can reduce anxiety-like behaviors in animal models and humans by influencing the GABA receptor system, which is responsible for regulating mood.

2. **Bifidobacterium longum (35624):** Research suggests that Bifidobacterium longum can improve mood and reduce anxiety by enhancing the production of neurotransmitters like serotonin, which is closely linked to mood regulation.

3. **Lactobacillus helveticus R0052 and Bifidobacterium longum R0175:** This combination of probiotics has been found to reduce anxiety symptoms in clinical studies, possibly through reducing levels of cortisol (the stress hormone) and improving the balance of gut microbiota.

4. **Lactobacillus acidophilus:** Some studies indicate that Lactobacillus acidophilus has a role in the production of neurotransmitters, including serotonin, and may help reduce anxiety by improving gut health.

5. **Bifidobacterium bifidum** is another strain that has been shown to

modulate the gut-brain axis, and some research has indicated that it can help alleviate symptoms of anxiety and depression.

6. Saccharomyces boulardii: This probiotic yeast has shown promise in reducing gut inflammation, which may, in turn, help improve mood and reduce anxiety symptoms by influencing the gut-brain connection.

7. Lactobacillus casei: Lactobacillus casei is another probiotic strain that has been studied for its calming effects, particularly for individuals experiencing stress and anxiety.

Evidence-Based Anxiety Management for Mothers

For mothers, particularly those recovering from postnatal depletion, these evidence-based techniques can help reduce anxiety:

1. **Mindful Breathing:** Encourages focus on the present, reducing racing thoughts and calming the mind.
2. **Cognitive Reframing:** Helps challenge and replace anxious thoughts with balanced perspectives.
3. **Structured Routines:** Creates predictability, minimizing feelings of chaos or uncertainty.
4. **Importance of Sunlight & Nature for Mental Health:** Exposure to sunlight and time spent in nature can profoundly impact mental health. Sunlight helps regulate circadian rhythms and boost mood through the production of serotonin and vitamin D. Aim to spend time outdoors each day, even if it's just a short walk or sitting in a sunlit area. Connecting with nature can also be therapeutic, reducing stress and enhancing feelings of well-being. Natural environments have been shown to improve mood, increase energy levels, and support overall mental health.
5. **Gentle exercise:** Gentle exercise such as walking outside increases endorphins, the body's natural mood boosters, which help reduce anxiety and stress and encourages the release of serotonin and dopamine, neu-

rotransmitters that promote feelings of well-being. Light movement helps regulate cortisol levels, preventing excessive stress buildup.

The Path Forward

Anxiety in mothers is common - but it's not inevitable, and it's not something you have to face alone. By combining practical support, professional help, and targeted lifestyle strategies, mothers can reduce the mental health toll of parenting and nurture both themselves and their families. Small changes in diet, rest, exercise, connection and other lifestyle changes can make a significant difference over time for a number of people.

9

Strategies for Sleep Struggles

The joy of welcoming a new baby often comes hand-in-hand with sleepless nights and overwhelming fatigue. A staggering 80% of new mothers report experiencing sleep disturbances in the first few months postpartum. However, the challenges of sleep can extend far beyond the initial weeks of motherhood, impacting women for years after giving birth. The term "tired but wired" aptly describes the conflicting feelings of exhaustion and restlessness many mothers face. This phenomenon can be attributed to a complex interplay of hormonal changes, lifestyle factors, and psychological stressors that significantly disrupt sleep patterns.

Insomnia is a common issue, affecting about one in three adults regularly. It is diagnosed when someone struggles to sleep for at least three nights a week for three months or more. For postnatally depleted women, the risk of insomnia can be even higher due to the physiological, hormonal, and emotional changes that occur after childbirth. Women who are postnatally depleted experience exhaustion from pregnancy and childbirth, combined with disrupted sleep from caring for a newborn. This depletion, along with fluctuating hormone levels, can affect their ability to get restful sleep, making them more prone to insomnia.

When a new mother is sleep-deprived, her memory, attention span, and decision-making abilities can suffer. Many doctors may not address this condition properly, even though chronic sleep deprivation can lead to significant long-term health problems, especially for postnatally depleted women. Some of the consequences include:

- **Slower reaction times**, making one more prone to accidents.
- **Decreased work and study performance**, with cognitive functions impaired by lack of sleep.
- **Unhealthy eating habits**, where fatigue causes cravings for quick, unhealthy foods that can harm gut health, lead to weight gain, and hinder overall recovery.
- **Increased physical health risks**, such as a heightened likelihood of developing diabetes, digestive disorders, and heart disease. Lack of sleep also elevates blood pressure, causes inflammation, and triggers the body's stress response system.
- **Mental health decline**, with insufficient sleep damaging brain health and increasing the risk of developing neurological and psychiatric conditions, such as postpartum depression.

Research indicates that those with poor physical, mental, and metabolic health are more likely to suffer from insomnia, which explains why postnatally depleted women – often juggling physical recovery, emotional stress, and newborn care – are more vulnerable to sleep disturbances.

For these women, prioritizing sleep is essential to recovery yet can be incredibly challenging. It may be helpful to explore natural remedies, such as supplements like magnesium, which can promote relaxation, or lifestyle changes like maintaining a consistent sleep routine, reducing screen time before bed, and incorporating calming activities, such as light yoga or meditation, before sleeping.

Hormonal Changes

One of the most significant contributors to sleep issues in new mothers besides the baby waking in the night is the dramatic shift in hormones following childbirth. After giving birth, levels of estrogen and progesterone plummet, which can lead to mood swings and fatigue. Additionally, postpartum mothers often experience fluctuating levels of cortisol, the body's primary stress hormone. Chronic stress from the demands of caring for a newborn can elevate cortisol levels, making it difficult to relax and fall asleep.

Thyroid function is another critical factor. Conditions such as postpartum thyroiditis can affect energy levels and mood, leading to symptoms of fatigue and anxiety. Prolactin, a hormone essential for milk production, can also impact sleep. Higher levels of prolactin in breastfeeding mothers may interfere with their ability to achieve restorative sleep, further contributing to feelings of being "wired."

Lifestyle Factors

The disruption of sleep due to a newborn's erratic schedule is perhaps the most recognizable challenge for new mothers. Frequent wake-ups for feedings, diaper changes, and comforting can lead to significant sleep deprivation, a problem that persists even as the child grows. Beyond the demands of parenting, environmental factors such as noise, light, and lack of personal space can further impede sleep quality.

Psychological factors play a substantial role in sleep disturbances as well. Many mothers experience postpartum anxiety and depression, which can exacerbate sleep problems. Research indicates that anxiety often manifests as a difficulty in unwinding, making it challenging to fall asleep at night. Additionally, the mental load of parenting—balancing schedules, managing household tasks, and worrying about the child – can keep mothers awake, perpetuating the cycle of fatigue and restlessness.

How to Improve Your Sleep

Improving sleep involves creating a conducive environment, adopting healthy habits, and addressing underlying issues. Here are 18 evidence-based tips to enhance your sleep quality:

- **Getting morning sunlight on your skin**: this helps your body adjust to the day and night cycle
- **Yoga stretches**: Stretching relaxes your muscles and makes you more comfortable before bed. I like to use YouTube for instant free classes; there are 1000's of videos to choose from.
- **Removing Sunglasses**: this might be hard for some people, but sunglasses can trick your body into thinking it's dark when it's not and disrupt your circadian rhythm.
- **Avoiding Food 3 hours Before Bed**: studies show that eating close to bedtime can interfere with your sleep. This might be because your body is busy digesting food.
- **Exercising in the Morning**: this boosts your natural melatonin production, which is a hormone that regulates your sleep. Modern life can make us less active than our ancestors, so we need to move more.
- **Dimming the lights**: turn your phone light on night mode and lower the brightness of your lights 2 hours before bed. Ideally, you should avoid screens 2 hours before bed, but I know that's not realistic for everyone.
- **Stick to a Sleep Schedule**: Go to bed and wake up at the same time every day, even on weekends. Consistency reinforces your circadian rhythm, making it easier to fall asleep and wake up naturally.
- **Optimize Your Sleep Environment**: Keep your bedroom dark, quiet, and cool (around 60–67°F or 16–19°C), invest in a comfortable mattress and pillows, consider blackout curtains or a white noise machine.
- **Limit Screen Time Before Bed**: The blue light emitted by phones, tablets, and TVs interferes with melatonin production. Avoid screens at least an hour before bedtime or use blue-light-blocking glasses.
- **Limit Alcohol Intake**: While alcohol may initially make you feel sleepy,

it can disrupt your sleep cycle and reduce the quality of deep sleep.
- **Manage Stress and Anxiety:** Practice mindfulness, meditation, or deep-breathing exercises to reduce stress and calm your mind before bed. Journaling can also help offload worries.
- **Avoid Heavy Meals Before Bed:** Eating large or spicy meals close to bedtime can cause indigestion, disrupting sleep. Opt for a light snack like a banana or a handful of nuts if you're hungry.
- **Limit Fluid Intake in the Evening:** Too many fluids can lead to frequent trips to the bathroom at night. Hydrate earlier in the day and reduce intake 2 hours before bed.
- **Use Aromatherapy:** Scents like lavender, chamomile, and cedarwood have calming properties. Use essential oils in a diffuser, pillow spray, or bath.
- **Prioritize Sleep**: Whenever possible, new mothers should take advantage of opportunities to nap when the baby sleeps, helping to mitigate sleep debt.
- **Establish a Routine**: Creating a consistent bedtime routine can signal to the body that it's time to wind down and prepare for sleep.
- **Mindfulness and Relaxation Techniques**: Incorporating practices such as mindfulness, meditation, or gentle yoga can help reduce stress levels and promote better sleep.
- **Seek Support**: Engaging with partners, family, or support groups can alleviate the mental load and provide emotional support, creating a more conducive environment for rest.

If you still have trouble sleeping after trying these things, it might indicate a deeper problem in your body. It could be related to high insulin levels, a lack of nutrients, an imbalance in your gut bacteria, a congested liver, hormonal issues, or a high level of toxins. You should see a doctor to rule out anything more serious.

Natural Herbs and Supplements to Support Sleep (with Breastfeeding Considerations)

Many natural remedies can help promote deeper, more restful sleep by easing stress, calming the nervous system, and supporting hormone balance. However, if you are breastfeeding, it's essential to approach herbs and supplements with caution - what you take may pass into your breast milk. Always check with a healthcare professional or lactation consultant before introducing any new supplement, especially while nursing.

Generally Considered Safe for Breastfeeding

Chamomile Tea

Chamomile is a gentle herbal tea traditionally used to calm the nervous system and ease digestion. It contains apigenin, an antioxidant that helps promote sleepiness by binding to calming receptors in the brain. In moderate amounts (e.g., 1–2 cups of tea per day), chamomile is generally considered safe while breastfeeding and can make a lovely bedtime ritual. However, monitor your baby for any sensitivity.

Magnesium (Glycinate or Citrate)

Magnesium is a vital mineral that helps relax muscles, calm the nervous system, and regulate neurotransmitters like GABA involved in sleep. Deficiencies are linked to insomnia, anxiety, and restlessness. Magnesium glycinate is a gentle, well-absorbed form often used to support sleep and stress resilience. It's considered safe for breastfeeding mothers and may even help ease muscle cramps or postpartum tension.

L-Theanine

Naturally found in green tea, L-theanine helps promote relaxation without drowsiness by increasing calming brain waves (alpha waves) and supporting GABA, serotonin, and dopamine levels. In supplement form, it's generally well tolerated and considered low risk, but still best to use with practitioner guidance while breastfeeding.

Glycine

Glycine is an amino acid that supports restful sleep by lowering body temperature and calming the nervous system. A small dose (around 3g) before bed has been shown to improve sleep quality and next-day alertness. It is naturally found in foods like bone broth and collagen, which are generally safe for breastfeeding and may be nourishing during postpartum recovery.

Use With Caution – Professional Guidance Advised

Reishi Mushroom (Ganoderma lucidum)

Reishi is an adaptogenic mushroom known for its calming and immune-supportive effects. While traditionally used to support sleep and reduce stress, limited safety data exists for use during breastfeeding. Speak with your practitioner or herbalist before use, especially if your baby is under 6 months or if you are on medication.

Niacinamide (Vitamin B3)

Niacinamide can support nervous system health and serotonin production and may help reduce restlessness. It is usually considered low-risk at moderate doses, but as with any supplement, consult your healthcare provider for appropriate dosing if breastfeeding.

Passionflower

Passionflower helps calm racing thoughts and supports GABA production. While it's often used in sleep blends, safety in breastfeeding is not well established, so it's best to avoid or use only with practitioner supervision.

Not Recommended While Breastfeeding

Valerian Root

Valerian is a potent herbal sedative. While effective for sleep in many adults, it is not considered safe during breastfeeding due to limited data and its strong effect on the nervous system. It may cause drowsiness in babies or alter their sleep patterns.

Adrenal Cortex Extracts

Supplements containing adrenal gland tissue (usually from bovine sources) are not recommended while breastfeeding due to potential hormonal effects and lack of safety data. Supporting adrenal health can be done through food, gentle stress management, and lifestyle strategies instead.

Ashwagandha

While often helpful for stress and cortisol balance, ashwagandha may not be appropriate during breastfeeding, particularly in large doses. It can have hormonal effects and is best avoided unless recommended by a knowledgeable practitioner.

Melatonin

Melatonin is a hormone naturally produced by the body to regulate sleep-wake cycles. It is also a powerful antioxidant that can protect cells from damage and reduce inflammation. Although available over the counter, melatonin supplements are not routinely recommended while breastfeeding, as the effects on infants and milk production are still not fully understood.

10

The Role of Exercise in Postpartum Recovery

Exercise offers a wide range of benefits that go far beyond weight loss or physical appearance. For postpartum mothers, gentle, consistent movement can be profoundly healing — supporting not only physical recovery, but also emotional well-being, hormone balance, and gut health. In a time marked by exhaustion, hormone shifts, and mental fog, exercise becomes less about performance and more about restoration.

Exercise for Mental Clarity and Emotional Well-being

One of the most immediate and noticeable benefits of movement is its effect on the mind. Postnatal life can bring feelings of overwhelm, anxiety, or "brain fog" — but regular physical activity has been shown to enhance mental clarity and emotional stability.

Exercise increases the production of endorphins, the body's natural mood boosters, which help reduce stress and improve overall outlook. It also promotes *neuroplasticity* — the brain's ability to adapt, reorganize, and form new neural connections. This means that even gentle movement can support better memory, focus, and resilience, helping mothers feel more present, grounded, and capable in their daily lives.

Supporting Hormonal Balance Through Movement

After childbirth, the body undergoes dramatic hormonal shifts. Levels of cortisol (the stress hormone) and insulin can fluctuate significantly, contributing to fatigue, irritability, and energy crashes. Exercise plays a key role in helping regulate these hormones.

By stabilizing blood sugar levels and reducing cortisol, movement can improve mood and boost overall energy. These effects aren't limited to high-intensity workouts — in fact, moderate and consistent activity is often more effective during this phase. Think of exercise as a gentle tool for rebalancing your internal systems, not something that needs to be intense or exhausting to be worthwhile.

Movement for Gut Health and Whole-Body Vitality

Emerging research shows that physical activity also plays a surprising role in gut health. Gentle exercise supports digestion, enhances immune function, and helps maintain a healthy gut microbiome — the community of bacteria that influences everything from mood to nutrient absorption.

Movement has been shown to increase the production of short-chain fatty acids and encourage the growth of beneficial gut bacteria. A thriving gut microbiome is especially important during the postpartum period, as it influences immune recovery, inflammation, and even the production of neurotransmitters that regulate mood.

That said, more isn't always better. Excessive or high-intensity training, especially without proper rest, can lead to "leaky gut" — a condition where the gut lining becomes more permeable, potentially increasing inflammation. It can also place extra strain on the adrenal glands, intensifying the fatigue many new mothers already feel.

Finding the Right Balance

The key is to approach movement with compassion. You don't need to push your limits — you need to support your recovery. Whether it's a short walk outside, a gentle yoga session, or simply stretching between feeds, what matters is that you're moving in ways that feel restorative, not depleting.

In the following section, we'll look at exactly how to get started — with safe, simple exercises that build strength, boost energy, and help you reconnect with your body.

Getting Started: Gentle Exercise for Postnatal Recovery

If you're feeling exhausted, run down, or unsure where to begin, take a deep breath. You don't need to jump into intense workouts, especially if you're just getting started — in fact, the best place to start is with gentle, manageable movement that supports your recovery without draining your energy.

A simple daily walk is one of the most effective and accessible ways to begin. Just stepping outside for fresh air and sunlight can help regulate your sleep, boost your mood, and restore energy levels. Even ten minutes can offer a sense of accomplishment — a small but powerful act of self-care during the early postpartum weeks.

When you're ready for more, start introducing low-impact exercises that rebuild strength safely and support your changing body. The focus at this stage should be on improving circulation, restoring core stability, and strengthening muscles that may have weakened during pregnancy and childbirth.

Try including the following in your weekly routine:

- **Walking**: Low-impact, easy to fit into your day, and great for cardiovascular health, circulation, and mood.
- **Pelvic Floor Exercises (Kegels)**: Essential for rebuilding internal support and bladder control.

- **Gentle Yoga or Stretching**: Eases tension, improves flexibility, and encourages relaxation.
- **Postnatal Pilates**: Supports core strength, spinal alignment, and pelvic stability.
- **Bodyweight Exercises**: Modified squats, lunges, and push-ups help rebuild muscle tone at your own pace.
- **Swimming or Water Aerobics**: Gentle on joints while offering full-body resistance training.
- **Breath Work & Core Activation**: Diaphragmatic breathing and deep core exercises (like engaging the transverse abdominis) help reconnect you to your body's foundation.
- **Light Strength Training**: Using resistance bands or light weights gradually rebuilds muscle tone and metabolism.

If time feels scarce (and let's be real — it often is), don't underestimate the value of short, consistent movement. Free online workouts — especially on platforms like YouTube — offer bite-sized sessions that fit into even the busiest days. Just a few minutes here and there can build momentum over time.

Remember, recovery isn't a race. Be kind to yourself, listen to your body, and move in ways that feel nourishing.

II

Part Two

As you move beyond the intensity of the first year—the sleepless nights, the hormone shifts, the steep learning curve—and begin to find your rhythm, this next stage offers a powerful opportunity to elevate your health to the next level. With breastfeeding behind you and babyhood giving way to toddlerhood, life starts to feel a little more spacious. It's time to step into a new chapter feeling stronger, clearer and more empowered than ever.

11

Balancing Hormones After the First Year

You made it through the sleepless nights, the early milestones, and maybe even returned to work — but something still feels off. Fatigue lingers, even when your little one sleeps through the night. Mood swings feel unfamiliar. Your periods may be irregular, your libido low, and your body harder to recognize. Hair may be thinning, weight clings on stubbornly, or you just don't feel like *yourself*.

These symptoms are common, but they're not something you just have to live with. More often than not, they're signs of deeper hormonal imbalances that haven't fully resolved since giving birth.

After childbirth, your body experiences one of the most intense hormonal shifts of a woman's lifetime. While some recalibration happens naturally in the early months, many mothers are left in a prolonged state of imbalance — especially when the demands of modern life, stress, poor sleep, and environmental toxins continue to interfere.

In fact, hormone-related conditions like PCOS, thyroid dysfunction, infertility, early puberty, and estrogen-driven cancers have risen sharply in recent decades. Researchers point to a mix of environmental chemicals, nutrient-depleted diets, stress, sleep loss, and lifestyle factors — all of which can delay recovery and make it harder for mothers to return to balance after birth.

In this chapter, we'll explore what healthy hormone recovery really looks like after the first year of motherhood, what symptoms to watch for, and how to gently support your body in finding its rhythm again — no matter how long it's been.

Why Are Hormones Still Out of Balance After the First Year of Motherhood?

Many women expect to feel "back to normal" a year after giving birth. But for a growing number of mothers, symptoms like fatigue, brain fog, low libido, anxiety, irregular periods, or stubborn weight gain don't disappear — and in some cases, they only *begin* after the first year.

The truth is, hormonal balance doesn't automatically return just because your baby turns one. In fact, the ongoing demands of motherhood, combined with modern stressors, can push the body into a state of chronic imbalance that lasts well into the toddler years — or longer — if not addressed.

Here are some of the key reasons hormonal recovery is so disrupted in today's world:

1. Environmental Endocrine Disruptors (EDCs)

From hormone-disrupting chemicals in plastics to phthalates in personal care products and pesticides in non-organic food, our bodies are constantly exposed to substances that mimic or block estrogen, testosterone, and thyroid hormones. These compounds interfere with natural hormone signaling — and when your body is already stretched thin from postnatal depletion, the impact can be even greater. This ongoing exposure can lead to symptoms like PMS, low libido, irritability, irregular cycles, or worsened postnatal anxiety — even long after your baby is out of nappies.

2. Processed Diets & Insulin Resistance

The typical modern diet — high in sugar, processed carbs, caffeine, and inflammatory fats — plays a big role in hormonal dysregulation. It contributes to blood sugar instability and insulin resistance, which can lead to estrogen dominance, fatigue, irritability, and fat storage around the belly. Even mothers who "eat well" may not be getting the nutrients required to support stable hormones — especially if they're still skipping meals, snacking in a rush, or relying on quick convenience foods between naps and school runs.

3. Chronic Stress & Sleep Deprivation

The first year of motherhood is intense, but the stress doesn't stop at 12 months. Toddlers bring a new level of unpredictability — and many mothers are also navigating work, relationships, and family logistics with little recovery time. Chronic stress increases cortisol, which disrupts thyroid function, suppresses progesterone, and makes you more prone to anxiety, burnout, PMS, and thyroid issues. Even if your baby sleeps better, you may not be getting the deep, restorative rest your hormones need to regulate.

4. Suboptimal Liver Function

The liver plays a vital role in detoxifying excess estrogen and other hormones. But when it's overburdened — from environmental toxins, alcohol, medication, nutrient deficiencies, or poor digestion — hormones are recycled instead of excreted. This can lead to bloating, mood swings, sore breasts, and heavy or painful periods. Many mothers unknowingly struggle with sluggish liver function that worsens over time, especially if they're relying on caffeine, skipping meals, or haven't restored nutrient stores post-birth.

5. Nutrient Depletion from Pregnancy & Breastfeeding

It takes years — not months — to replenish the nutrients lost through pregnancy, birth, and breastfeeding. Key vitamins and minerals like iron, magnesium, zinc, B vitamins, and omega-3s are essential for hormone production and balance. If those stores aren't fully restored, it can impair thyroid function, disrupt ovulation, increase anxiety or depression, and prolong postnatal depletion. Many mothers are unknowingly running on empty — long after the baby phase is over.

6. Gut Health and Hormone Metabolism

Your gut isn't just for digestion, it plays a crucial role in metabolizing hormones, especially estrogen. Inside your gut lives a subset of bacteria called the estrobolome, which helps regulate how much estrogen is reabsorbed or eliminated from the body. When your microbiome is imbalanced (a condition called dysbiosis), excess estrogen can recirculate, leading to symptoms like bloating, mood swings, heavy periods, and hormonal acne.

After pregnancy and breastfeeding — especially if you've had antibiotics, birth interventions, processed foods, or stress — your gut barrier and microbial diversity may be compromised. This affects not only hormone clearance but also your ability to absorb the key nutrients (like zinc, B vitamins, and magnesium) needed to make and regulate hormones in the first place.

An unhealthy gut can quietly sabotage hormonal recovery for years, contributing to fatigue, skin issues, anxiety, and ongoing PMS — long after the fourth trimester is over.

7. Better Awareness and Diagnosis

The rise in hormone-related conditions isn't only due to external factors, they are also more likely to be identifed. Disorders like PCOS, thyroid dysfunction, and endometriosis, once dismissed or overlooked, are finally getting more attention. This means more mothers are being diagnosed *after* the first year, when persistent symptoms prompt further investigation. Recognition is the first step — but many women still struggle to get the support and treatment they need.

Nourishing Your Hormones

After the first intense year of motherhood — when your body is no longer sustaining another life through pregnancy or breastfeeding — it's finally time to turn your attention inward. But for many mothers, lingering symptoms like mood swings, anxiety, stubborn weight, fatigue, or irregular periods are a sign that your hormones are still out of balance.

The truth is, food can be one of your greatest allies in rebalancing your hormones after the rollercoaster of pregnancy and postpartum. Women's hormones, including estrogen, progesterone, cortisol, insulin and thyroid hormones — are incredibly sensitive to what we eat. The nutrients (or lack thereof) in your diet influence how these hormones are made, how they function, how they're cleared from your body, and how they interact with your brain, metabolism, and reproductive system.

It's estimated that up to 80% of women experience hormone-related issues at some point and yet many are told it's just a "normal" part of womanhood. But feeling overwhelmed, exhausted, or inflamed doesn't have to be your new normal.

Let's explore the foods and products that support, disrupt, or sabotage hormonal healing.

The Good: Hormone-Supportive Foods

The right foods provide the raw materials your body needs to create and regulate hormones effectively. Here's what to prioritise:

Healthy Fats

Your reproductive hormones — estrogen, progesterone, testosterone, and cortisol — are made from cholesterol. Healthy fat intake is essential for producing and regulating these and other hormones. That means dietary fat isn't the enemy; it's a necessity. Healthy fats like avocado, oily fish, eggs, coconut, nuts, seeds, ghee, and extra virgin olive oil support hormone production, reduce inflammation, and stabilise blood sugar — all essential for emotional and physical balance.

Omega-3 fatty acids, found in fatty fish (like salmon, sardines, and mackerel), flaxseed, and chia seeds, are particularly powerful for reducing menstrual pain, easing anxiety, and supporting cortisol regulation.

Fibre-Rich Foods

Fibre helps your body eliminate excess estrogen via the digestive tract. Without enough fibre, estrogen can recirculate and lead to symptoms of estrogen dominance — like PMS, mood swings, bloating, and breast tenderness.

Support your gut-liver-hormone axis with fibre-rich foods like leafy greens, legumes, flaxseeds, pears, avocados, lentils, raspberries, chickpeas, and artichokes.

Cruciferous Vegetables

Broccoli, kale, cauliflower, and Brussels sprouts contain a compound called indole-3-carbinol, which helps the liver metabolize estrogen more efficiently. These detox-friendly vegetables are linked to a reduced risk of hormone-sensitive conditions like endometriosis and breast cancer.

Fermented Foods

Gut health is directly linked to hormone health. A healthy microbiome helps metabolize estrogen, supports mood, and boosts nutrient absorption. Add probiotic-rich foods like yogurt, kefir, sauerkraut, kimchi, and miso to support digestion and hormonal regulation.

Protein & Amino Acids

Protein provides the building blocks for many hormones. Tyrosine supports thyroid function and dopamine production, while tryptophan supports serotonin — crucial for mood and sleep. Eggs, turkey, nuts, seeds, legumes, and fish are excellent postpartum staples.

The Bad: Hormone-Disrupting Foods

Certain common foods can throw hormones out of balance by affecting insulin, cortisol, or estrogen levels. These include:

Refined Carbohydrates & Sugars
Excess sugar leads to insulin spikes, which drive inflammation and fat storage. Over time, this can contribute to insulin resistance — a key driver of hormonal issues like PCOS. Sugar also raises cortisol, your stress hormone, leading to fatigue, cravings, anxiety, and poor sleep.

Conventional Meat & Dairy
Non-organic animal products may contain added hormones and antibiotics that interfere with your own hormonal balance. These additives can mimic estrogen in the body and worsen conditions like fibroids, PMS, or hormonal acne. When possible, choose organic, grass-fed, hormone-free options.

Alcohol
Even moderate alcohol intake can disrupt liver function, impair hormone clearance, and increase circulating estrogen. In women, this raises the risk of PMS, fibroids, fertility issues, and breast cancer. Reducing or eliminating alcohol is one of the most powerful ways to support long-term hormone health.

The Ugly: Toxins and Ultra-Processed Foods

Some of the worst offenders for hormonal health come in the form of chemicals, fake ingredients, and industrialized packaging:

Ultra-Processed Foods
Highly processed foods — think packaged snacks, sugary cereals, fast food, soft drinks — contain a cocktail of additives, trans fats, and preservatives

that wreak havoc on your endocrine system. These foods drive inflammation, dysregulate insulin, and offer no nutritional support for hormone production.

Endocrine-Disrupting Chemicals (EDCs)

These are synthetic compounds that mimic or block hormones in the body — especially estrogen. Common EDCs like BPA and phthalates are found in plastic containers, canned food linings, cosmetics, cleaning products, and pesticides. Long-term exposure has been linked to infertility, PCOS, thyroid dysfunction, and early puberty.

Support your body by:

- Avoiding plastic food storage and drink bottles
- Choosing organic produce when possible
- Limiting canned foods and processed snacks
- Using natural personal care products

Vitamins & Minerals that Nourish Hormones

Beyond whole foods, specific nutrients play key roles in hormone synthesis and balance. Here's what to focus on:

B Vitamins

B6, B12 and folate (B9) support neurotransmitters like serotonin and dopamine and help regulate insulin. B vitamin-rich foods (leafy greens, liver, eggs, legumes, meats) are especially important for energy and mood stability in motherhood.

Vitamin D

This vitamin is a precursor to several hormones and supports thyroid, bone, and immune function. Low levels are linked to mood disorders and hormone imbalances. Get 10–20 minutes of sunlight daily and consider supplementation along with vitamin K if levels are low.

Thyroid-Supportive Minerals

- **Iodine**: For thyroid hormone production (found in seaweed, eggs, iodised salt)
- **Selenium**: Converts T4 to active T3 (found in Brazil nuts, eggs, tuna)
- **Zinc**: Supports hormone receptor function (found in oysters, pumpkin seeds, red meat)

Final Thought

As you can see, postnatal hormone imbalance isn't just about getting older or being a tired mum — it's a complex web of modern-day stressors, nutrient needs, and physiological shifts that require time, nourishment, and support to fully recover from.

Hormone Restoration Meal Plan

This one-week meal plan is designed to help restore and rebalance your hormones beyond the first year of motherhood. It's simple, delicious, and built around real food that supports energy, mood, metabolism, and menstrual health.

Every day includes complete protein, healthy fats, and a wide variety of vegetables, herbs and hormone-supportive ingredients. Meals are nutrient-dense, gut-friendly, and anti-inflammatory — without being expensive, complicated, or restrictive.

You'll see ingredients repeated across the week in smart ways, so you can prep once and eat twice. The goal isn't perfection — it's to make hormone restoration practical, doable, and nourishing for real life.

Day 1

- **Breakfast**: Avocado and smoked salmon on whole-grain toast with spinach and a sprinkle of flaxseeds for omega-3.
- **Lunch**: Mixed greens salad with grilled chicken, pumpkin seeds, carrots, red bell pepper, cucumber, and olive oil vinaigrette.
- Snack: Coconut yogurt with a handful of berries and a drizzle of honey.
- **Dinner**: Baked salmon with quinoa, steamed broccoli, and a side of roasted sweet potato.

Day 2

- **Breakfast**: Smoothie with organic soy milk, spinach, frozen banana, flax seeds, 2 medjool dates, and protein powder.
- **Lunch**: Chickpea and organic tofu with chicken and vegetable stir-fry with bell peppers, zucchini, carrots, and a sesame-tahini dressing.
- **Snack**: Apple slices with almond butter.
- **Dinner**: Grass-fed beef stir-fry with brown rice, Bok choy, mushrooms, and ginger.

Day 3

- **Breakfast**: Whole organic oats with walnuts, chia seeds, sliced apple, and a sprinkle of cinnamon.
- **Lunch**: Lentil and vegetable soup (carrots, celery, garlic, onions, sweet potato and spinach) with preservative (nitrate) free bacon, a slice of sourdough toast.
- **Snack**: Handful of mixed nuts (walnuts, almonds, and Brazil nuts for selenium).
- **Dinner**: Grilled chicken with mashed cauliflower, green beans, and a

side of roasted Brussels sprouts.

Day 4

- **Breakfast**: Veggie egg omelet with spinach, bell peppers, tomatoes, and a sprinkle of goat cheese, served with a side of avocado.
- **Lunch**: Sardines, avocado lettuce, cucumber, beetroot and shredded carrots sandwich on traditional sourdough bread
- **Snack**: Cottage cheese with sliced strawberries.
- **Dinner**: Prawn and veggie stir-fry with asparagus, red cabbage, and cauliflower rice, topped with a sprinkle of sesame seeds.

Day 5

- **Breakfast**: Chia pudding (prepared the night before with organic soy milk and chia seeds) topped with fresh berries and a spoonful of almond butter.
- **Lunch**: Quinoa bowl with black beans, avocado, shredded kale, roasted sweet potato, and a lemon-tahini dressing.
- **Snack**: Celery sticks with hummus.
- **Dinner**: Baked chicken thighs with roasted butternut squash and broccoli with grass-fed butter

Day 6

- **Breakfast**: Smoothie bowl with spinach, banana, frozen berries, and a topping of hemp seeds, flax seeds, and a few pumpkin seeds.
- **Lunch**: Tuna salad on a bed of mixed greens with beetroot, cucumber, olives, cherry tomatoes, and a drizzle of olive oil and balsamic vinegar.
- **Snack**: Carrot sticks with guacamole.
- **Dinner**: Zucchini noodles with grass-fed beef meatballs, marinara sauce, and a side of sautéed spinach.

Day 7

- **Breakfast**: 3 scrambled eggs with turmeric, spinach, onion, cherry tomatoes, and a side of sourdough toast.
- **Lunch**: Grilled salmon salad with arugula, avocado, shredded carrots, sunflower seeds, and lemon-olive oil dressing.
- **Snack**: Handful of trail mix with nuts and seeds (avoid added sugars).
- **Dinner**: Stuffed bell peppers with quinoa, black beans, diced tomatoes, onions, and a sprinkle of cheese (optional), served with a grass-fed steak

Key Hormone-Supportive Elements in This Plan

Hormone-Balancing Fats

- **Avocados, olive oil, coconut oil, olives, and fatty fish** provide essential fats that support hormone synthesis and reduce inflammation.
- **Omega-3s** (from salmon, sardines, flaxseeds, and walnuts) help regulate estrogen, improve mood, and reduce period pain.

High-Quality Protein

- Each meal includes complete protein sources (chicken, eggs, tofu, fish, beef, or protein powder) to stabilize blood sugar and support hormone production.
- Legumes like lentils and chickpeas add plant-based variety and fiber.

Complex Carbohydrates & Fiber

- **Quinoa, sweet potato, oats, brown rice, and flaxseeds** support steady energy and hormone detoxification via the gut.
- **Fiber** helps remove excess estrogen through improved bowel function.

Micronutrients for Hormonal Health

- **Magnesium** (from quinoa, leafy greens, and pumpkin seeds) supports sleep and adrenal function. .
- **Zinc** (from beef, pumpkin seeds) aids in progesterone and thyroid hormone production.
- **Selenium** (from Brazil nuts, fish) supports thyroid health.
- **B vitamins** (from eggs, meat, leafy greens) are vital for mood and metabolism.
- **Vitamin D** (from salmon, eggs, or fortified options) supports immune and hormone regulation.

Gut & Liver Support

- **Fermented foods** (coconut yogurt, pickles) and high-fiber veggies support gut health and estrogen clearance.
- **Liver-supportive foods** like leafy greens, lemon, and cruciferous vegetables help metabolize and eliminate used hormones.

Blood Sugar Stability

- Regular protein, paired with **complex carbs and healthy fats**, prevents blood sugar spikes — reducing cortisol, insulin resistance, and mood swings.

Low in Inflammatory Foods

- This plan minimizes **refined sugar, seed oils, gluten, and dairy** — common hormone disruptors and inflammation triggers, especially in sensitive individuals.

12

Stress Less by Controlling Cortisol

Cortisol is your body's built-in alarm system. Known as the "stress hormone," it helps you wake up, manage your energy, regulate inflammation, balance blood sugar, and respond to life's demands. In the short term, cortisol is essential. But when it stays elevated for too long — as it often does in modern motherhood — it can quietly sabotage your health.

After the first year of motherhood, many women expect to feel more like themselves again. But instead, they're still running on adrenaline: juggling toddlers, work, household pressures, emotional load, and sleepless nights. This chronic, low-grade stress keeps cortisol levels high — and over time, this "silent stress" can take a toll on your mood, hormones, metabolism, and immune system.

Could Your Cortisol Be Too High?

Cortisol dysfunction is one of the most under-recognized issues among mothers — and it doesn't always show up as obvious stress. You might be smiling on the outside, but inside, your body is struggling to regulate and recover.

Common signs of elevated cortisol include:

- Feeling wired but tired
- Trouble falling or staying asleep
- Sugar or salt cravings
- Weight gain around the middle
- Anxiety, overwhelm, or irritability
- Frequent colds or slow healing
- Brain fog or poor memory
- Low libido
- Irregular or painful periods
- Hair thinning or breakage
- Feeling "on edge" or emotionally fragile

If you're nodding yes to several of these, your body may be stuck in a state of chronic stress — even if you're powering through the day.

Why High Cortisol Is Harmful

When cortisol remains high for months or even years, it disrupts many essential systems:

- **Hormones**: It can lower progesterone and thyroid hormones, contributing to PMS, irregular cycles, fatigue, and infertility.
- **Immunity**: It suppresses immune function, making you more prone to getting sick or staying sick.
- **Metabolism**: It increases insulin resistance, blood sugar issues, and abdominal fat storage.
- **Mood**: It's linked to anxiety, depression, irritability, and burnout.

With over 75% of adults reporting moderate to high stress and nearly half saying their stress has increased, managing cortisol is no longer a luxury — it's a health necessity.

Natural Ways to Reduce Cortisol

The good news? You can lower your cortisol levels through practical lifestyle shifts. Small daily changes add up to big improvements in your energy, clarity, and emotional resilience.

1. Eat to Balance Blood Sugar and Support Stress Resilience

Cortisol is closely linked to blood sugar stability. Skipping meals, relying on caffeine, or eating processed snacks can spike blood sugar — and cortisol follows. The solution? Eat balanced meals with **protein, fiber, healthy fats**, and slow-burning carbs.

Key nutrients that help reduce cortisol include:

- **Omega-3s** (salmon, flaxseeds, walnuts): Reduce inflammation and blunt cortisol spikes
- **Magnesium** (leafy greens, pumpkin seeds, dark chocolate): Supports calm, sleep, and adrenal recovery
- **B vitamins** (meat, eggs, legumes, leafy greens): Needed for stress tolerance and hormone production

Tip: Build meals that include protein, colorful veggies, and a healthy fat source to help stabilize cortisol naturally.

2. Move Gently and Often

Exercise is a powerful way to regulate stress — but intensity matters. While high-intensity workouts can temporarily raise cortisol, regular **moderate movement** actually lowers your baseline levels.

Effective options include:

- Walking in nature
- Yoga or Pilates

- Swimming
- Dance or light strength training

A study found that people who exercised for 30 minutes a day had **25% lower cortisol** than those who were sedentary. Even 10-minute walks throughout your day can help reduce tension and reset your nervous system.

3. Practice Mindfulness and Deep Rest

Mindfulness practices like meditation, slow breathing, and gratitude journaling can train your brain to **calm the cortisol loop**. You don't need to sit cross-legged for an hour — just a few minutes of intentional stillness can make a difference.

- **Mindfulness-Based Stress Reduction (MBSR)** techniques have been shown to reduce cortisol by 15–20%.
- **Yoga** combines movement, breath, and mindfulness — studies show it can reduce cortisol by up to 30%.
- **Breathwork** activates the parasympathetic nervous system, your body's "rest and digest" mode.

Try: 4-7-8 breathing (inhale for 4 seconds, hold for 7, exhale for 8) — it's a powerful tool for calming the nervous system.

4. Prioritize Restorative Sleep

Sleep is one of the most effective ways to reset cortisol. But many mothers are chronically sleep-deprived — and that alone can keep cortisol levels elevated.

Aim for:

- 7–8 hours of **quality** sleep (even if broken, naps help)
- Consistent sleep and wake times

- A calming evening routine: dim lights, magnesium baths, screen-free wind-down time

Final Thoughts

High cortisol may be common, but it's not inevitable. You don't need to overhaul your life, choose one or two small ways to bring more nourishment, movement, calm and rest into your days.

13

When PMS Returns — Causes & Holistic Relief

The return of your period after having a baby can feel like a milestone — a sign your body is slowly finding its rhythm again. But when it's accompanied by mood swings, bloating, irritability, headaches, and unexpected emotional outbursts, it can also feel like a cruel twist of timing. You're likely still juggling disrupted sleep, an intense daily load, and possibly breastfeeding — so when PMS symptoms return in full force, it's no wonder many mothers feel confused, overwhelmed, or even betrayed by their own bodies.

PMS is common, affecting up to 75% of menstruating women, but after the first year of motherhood, it often hits differently — and sometimes more intensely. That's because your hormones are still recalibrating long after the newborn phase has passed. Estrogen and progesterone may remain out of balance, cycles may still be irregular, and nutrient depletion is still very real. Add chronic stress, overstimulation, and the emotional labor of modern motherhood to the mix — and your system is more sensitive to hormonal shifts than ever before.

For some mothers, PMS begins before their period even returns — showing up as irritability, low mood, or fatigue during the weeks before their first bleed. For others, periods return but feel unfamiliar, heavier, more painful, or emotionally turbulent. This often has less to do with age, and more to do with the cumulative effects of depletion, inflammation, stress, and unaddressed hormone imbalances that have quietly built up over the first year (or longer) of caring for a child.

In this chapter, we'll explore why PMS can worsen after childbirth — even after the so-called "fourth trimester" is over — and what you can do to support a smoother hormonal transition. We'll look at the deeper root causes behind PMS in the postnatal years and share nutrition, lifestyle, and functional tools that help ease symptoms naturally, so you can feel more like yourself again.

What Makes PMS Worse After Having a Baby?

1. Postpartum Hormone Fluctuations

Your hormones shift dramatically in the year after childbirth. Estrogen and progesterone, which surged during pregnancy, plummet after delivery. As your cycle resumes, these hormones can fluctuate wildly — leading to increased sensitivity to even minor changes. For women with underlying hormone imbalances (like estrogen dominance or low progesterone), PMS symptoms may feel worse than before pregnancy.

2. Depleted Nutrient Stores

Pregnancy, birth, and breastfeeding demand a lot from your body — especially your stores of magnesium, B vitamins, zinc, and omega-3s. These nutrients are critical for neurotransmitter balance, hormone metabolism, and nervous system health. If not replenished, deficiencies can amplify PMS symptoms like mood swings, anxiety, bloating, and sleep disturbances.

3. HPA Axis Dysregulation (Chronic Stress)

New motherhood is inherently stressful — even joyful stress still impacts your body. Cortisol, your main stress hormone, can interfere with progesterone production and hormone balance. When your body is chronically stressed, it prioritizes survival over reproduction, leading to irregular cycles and worsening PMS symptoms.

4. Gut-Hormone Connection

The gut microbiome plays a major role in hormone regulation. A group of gut bacteria known as the estrobolome helps metabolise and eliminate estrogen. When the gut is imbalanced (dysbiosis), estrogen may build up in the body, worsening PMS symptoms like bloating, breast tenderness, and mood swings.

5. Toxin Exposure

Endocrine-disrupting chemicals (EDCs), such as BPA and phthalates, can interfere with hormone signaling. These are commonly found in plastics, cosmetics, and non-organic produce. Minimizing exposure can support hormonal balance.

Functional Medicine Approach to Postpartum PMS

Functional medicine looks at PMS as the result of interconnected systems — not a standalone issue. Addressing the root causes of hormonal imbalance can bring relief.

Hormonal Imbalances and Estrogen Dominance

Women with heightened sensitivity to hormonal changes may experience more pronounced symptoms. Functional medicine often focuses on estrogen dominance — where estrogen levels are high relative to progesterone. This can worsen PMS symptoms such as mood swings, bloating, and breast tenderness. Supporting liver detoxification and gut health helps reduce excess estrogen.

Nutritional Deficiencies

Key nutrient shortfalls linked to PMS include magnesium, vitamin B6, calcium, and omega-3s. Magnesium helps regulate mood and muscle tension. B6 supports neurotransmitter production. Calcium stabilizes mood. Omega-3s reduce inflammation and support brain health. Replenishing these nutrients can significantly improve symptoms.

Stress and the HPA Axis

Chronic stress disrupts the HPA axis, leading to cortisol imbalances. Elevated cortisol interferes with hormonal signaling, intensifying PMS. Strategies to support stress resilience include mindfulness, gentle exercise, adaptogenic herbs (like ashwagandha and rhodiola), and sleep hygiene.

Gut Microbiome Health

Promote gut health with a high-fiber diet, fermented foods (like kefir and sauerkraut), and polyphenol-rich fruits and vegetables. This supports estrogen clearance and reduces inflammatory triggers of PMS.

Genetic and Epigenetic Factors

Genetic predispositions affect how your body processes hormones and neurotransmitters. For example, variations in genes involved in serotonin production or methylation (like MTHFR) can make PMS worse. Functional medicine can personalize care based on genetic and lifestyle factors.

Natural Remedies for PMS Relief

Consult a health practitioner before starting any new supplement regime, especially if still breastfeeding.

1. Anti-Inflammatory Diet: Your PMS Superpower

Eat plenty of fruits, vegetables, whole grains, nuts, seeds, and omega-3-rich foods like salmon. Add turmeric (curcumin) with black pepper for better absorption. These foods reduce inflammation, bloating, and mood swings.

2. St. John's Wort: Mood Booster

St. John's Wort influences serotonin levels and can ease mild PMS-related mood disturbances. Caution: It may interact with medications like birth control and antidepressants. Check with your healthcare provider.

3. Evening Primrose Oil: Hormonal Harmony

Rich in GLA (gamma-linolenic acid), this oil helps reduce breast tenderness and mood swings. Take 500–1,000 mg daily during the luteal phase for best results.

4. Heat Therapy

Place a hot water bottle on your lower abdomen for 20–30 minutes to ease cramps and relax muscles. Studies show heat therapy can be as effective as ibuprofen.

5. Walking: Gentle Movement for Relief

Regular movement increases endorphins and reduces PMS symptoms. A 20–30 minute walk three times a week during the luteal phase can help significantly.

6. Herbal Teas

- **Ginger:** Anti-inflammatory and pain relieving
- **Chamomile:** Calms the nervous system and promotes relaxation
- **Cinnamon:** Improves circulation and eases cramping

7. Magnesium: The PMS Mineral

Take 250–400 mg daily to relieve bloating, cramps, and mood swings. Use a high-quality magnesium glycinate supplement or add Epsom salt baths to your routine.

8. Vitamin B6: Mood Supporter

Supports serotonin production. Take 50–100 mg daily. Look for active (methylated) forms if you have the MTHFR gene variant. Include foods like bananas, poultry, and avocados.

9. Calcium: The Mood Stabiliser

Calcium supplementation has been shown to reduce mood swings, fatigue, and cravings. Aim for 1,000 mg daily through food or supplements. Leafy greens, dairy, or fortified plant milks are good sources.

Can You Get PMS While Breastfeeding?

Yes. Ovulation can occur before your first postpartum period. PMS symptoms may emerge even before menstruation returns. If you're feeling irritable, anxious, or unusually fatigued, it could be hormonal. Track your cycle, nourish your body, and consider natural supports. Your symptoms are valid — and manageable.

Final Thoughts

PMS symptoms may return more intensely than before, but they're not something you just have to put up with. By understanding the root causes and using targeted, natural strategies, you can find relief and feel more balanced in your body again. Support your hormones with nourishment, stress resilience, gut care and rest.

14

Health & Healing Begins in the Gut

The human body is a marvel of complexity, but it does not operate alone. It is home to trillions of microorganisms that collectively form the gut microbiome — an invisible ecosystem that influences nearly every system in the body. While most people associate the gut with digestion, the microbiome also plays critical roles in immunity, metabolism, mood, and hormonal balance — areas especially vital for women in the years following childbirth.

Recent research reveals that nurturing gut health is one of the most effective ways women can support healing and vitality beyond the first year of motherhood. By addressing imbalances through food, targeted supplements, stress reduction, and lifestyle shifts, we activate the body's innate capacity for self-repair and resilience. In many cases, the gut holds the key to resolving persistent health concerns.

Gut Health & Metabolism: More Than Just a Weight Issue

Gut microbes directly influence how our bodies store fat, regulate blood sugar, and use energy. In fact, imbalances in the gut microbiome are strongly associated with metabolic disorders such as obesity, type 2 diabetes, and polycystic ovary syndrome (PCOS).

For women, these aren't just cosmetic concerns. Obesity increases the risk of infertility, cardiovascular disease, hormone-related cancers, and early mortality. Research shows that women with obesity often have reduced microbial diversity and an overrepresentation of Firmicutes — bacteria linked to increased fat absorption and storage.

Even cravings may be influenced by your microbiome. Certain gut bacteria produce compounds that communicate with the brain's reward centers. For example, Firmicutes promote sugar cravings and satisfaction after carb-heavy meals, while Bacteroides — associated with lower BMI — may reduce sweet cravings. This opens the door for microbiome-targeted strategies that support appetite regulation and healthier food choices.

The Gut-Brain Connection: A New Lens on Mental Health

Anxiety, mood swings, and emotional exhaustion are all too common in the years after childbirth. The gut-brain axis — the communication network between your gut and central nervous system — plays a central role in regulating mood and mental well-being.

About 90% of the body's serotonin, a key mood-regulating neurotransmitter, is produced in the gut. A well-balanced microbiome helps regulate serotonin levels, while dysbiosis (gut imbalance) has been linked to anxiety and depression. For women navigating the hormonal fluctuations of motherhood, perimenopause, or stress, supporting gut health can provide emotional resilience and mental clarity.

Immunity Starts in the Gut

Nearly 70% of your immune system resides in the gut. The gut's immune tissues — particularly the gut-associated lymphoid tissue (GALT) — act as a first line of defense against pathogens.

The microbiome plays a crucial role in "training" immune cells to respond appropriately, reducing the risk of autoimmune conditions. This is especially relevant for women, who are disproportionately affected by autoimmune diseases like lupus, rheumatoid arthritis, and multiple sclerosis. Gut imbalances may contribute to the development or worsening of these conditions, making gut support a vital part of prevention and management.

Gut Health & Hormonal Balance: The Hidden Link

Hormones govern everything from your energy and mood to fertility and metabolism. And many of these hormones rely on a healthy gut for regulation. Let's explore how:

1. Estrogen Metabolism

Certain gut bacteria (especially Bifidobacterium and Lactobacillus) help metabolize and eliminate excess estrogen. When this process is disrupted, it can lead to estrogen dominance — a factor in PMS, fibroids, endometriosis, and hormone-sensitive cancers.

   A high-fiber diet supports these beneficial bacteria, naturally helping to keep estrogen levels balanced. Notably, up to 80% of women report PMS symptoms, and growing evidence suggests gut imbalances are part of the picture.

2. Thyroid Function

The gut also influences thyroid health by converting inactive T4 hormone into active T3. Gut dysbiosis and chronic inflammation can interfere with this process and suppress the hypothalamic-pituitary-thyroid (HPT) axis. Since around 60% of thyroid disease sufferers are women, the link between gut and thyroid cannot be overlooked.

3. Blood Sugar & Insulin Sensitivity

Gut bacteria help regulate insulin sensitivity and blood sugar levels. Imbalances, particularly an overgrowth of Firmicutes, may contribute to insulin resistance — a hallmark of type 2 diabetes and PCOS. A diverse gut microbiome supports more stable blood sugar and metabolic resilience.

4. Cortisol & the Stress Response

The gut also regulates how we respond to stress. Dysbiosis can disrupt the hypothalamic-pituitary-adrenal (HPA) axis, leading to elevated cortisol — the "stress hormone." Chronically high cortisol is linked to fatigue, poor sleep, anxiety, and menstrual disruptions. Supporting your gut can help restore hormonal rhythm and reduce the impact of stress.

Gut Health & Aging: What Changes and Why It Matters

As we age, gut health becomes more fragile. Microbial diversity — a hallmark of a healthy gut — tends to decline over time. This loss is associated with chronic inflammation, increased infections, and a higher risk of disease.

1. Digestion Slows Down

Stomach acid and digestive enzymes decline with age, reducing nutrient absorption. This can lead to deficiencies in vitamin B12, iron, and calcium — nutrients crucial for energy, mood, and bone health. Sluggish digestion may also cause bloating, gas, and discomfort.

2. Reduced Gut Motility

With age, food moves more slowly through the digestive tract, increasing the risk of constipation and bacterial imbalance. Longer transit time gives harmful microbes more opportunity to proliferate and disrupt the ecosystem.

3. Immune Decline (Immunosenescence)

The gut's immune function weakens with age, increasing vulnerability to infections, inflammation, and conditions like irritable bowel syndrome. This also raises the risk for inflammatory diseases and certain cancers.

The Consequences of Poor Gut Health

- **Chronic Inflammation**: Dysbiosis fuels persistent low-grade inflammation (known as "inflammaging"), which is linked to heart disease, diabetes, and cognitive decline.
- **Cognitive Decline**: Gut changes can impair neurotransmitter function, contributing to depression, memory loss, and conditions like Alzheimer's.
- **Nutrient Deficiencies**: Poor gut function impairs absorption of essential vitamins and minerals, impacting everything from bone density to brain health.
- **Skin Issues**: Conditions like acne, eczema, rosacea, and psoriasis have been linked to gut dysbiosis and inflammation, often referred to as the "gut-skin axis."

- **Increased Food Sensitivities**: An imbalanced gut can impair the intestinal lining (often called "leaky gut"), allowing undigested food particles to enter the bloodstream and triggering immune responses to certain foods.
- **Mood Instability & Irritability**: Disruptions in gut bacteria can interfere with neurotransmitter production, leading to increased irritability, mood swings, and emotional sensitivity.
- **Poor Detoxification**: The gut plays a major role in eliminating toxins and excess hormones. When the microbiome is out of balance, detox pathways become sluggish, increasing the body's toxic burden.

How to Support Your Gut (Now and Later)

Taking care of your gut is one of the most impactful health investments you can make as a woman and mother. Here's how:

- **Eat a fiber-rich diet**: Fruits, vegetables, whole grains, legumes, and seeds feed beneficial bacteria.
- **Include fermented foods**: Yogurt, kefir, sauerkraut, kimchi, and miso introduce healthy microbes.
- **Prioritize sleep and stress management**: Both play major roles in microbial balance.
- **Move your body daily**: Regular physical activity boosts gut motility and microbial diversity.
- **Use targeted supplements if needed**: Probiotics and prebiotics can help restore balance during periods of stress, illness, or antibiotic use.

Final Thoughts

The gut is not just the center of digestion — it's the command center for your metabolism, mood, hormones, and immune system. For mothers navigating the changes of postpartum life and beyond, prioritizing gut health can be transformative. It's a powerful reminder that healing, energy, and clarity often begin in the most unexpected place: the gut.

15

Gut Health Restoration - Remove, Replace, Repair, Restore Protocol

Integrative doctors and holistic health practitioners view a healthy gut as the cornerstone of vitality. When gut health falters, the ripple effects can touch nearly every system in the body. This is why the Four R Protocol – Remove, Replace, Repair, and Restore – is a transformative framework for those seeking to reclaim their health.

By addressing root causes and nourishing the gut, this protocol lays the foundation for enduring health and well-being. Whether you are managing chronic illness, enhancing resilience, or simply seeking to feel your best, the Three R approach offers a clear, evidence-based path forward. Here's a step-by-step approach to enhancing your gut health, based on current research in holistic nutrition and the gut microbiome.

NOTE BEFORE STARTING

This gut healing protocol should be followed under the guidance of an experienced practitioner and supported by appropriate testing (e.g., comprehensive stool testing, food sensitivity testing, SIBO breath tests, or organic acid testing). Each individual's gut health issues and needs will vary and personalized guidance is essential for best results and safety.

Step 1: Remove - Eliminating Gut Irritants

Duration: Maintain step 1 throughout all steps - the whole protocol - except for the pathogen removal which is between 2 to 6 weeks.

The first step in restoring gut health is identifying and removing irritants that disrupt the microbiome and trigger inflammation. Key culprits include:

1. **Remove Most Common Allergens:** Common triggers include gluten, dairy, soy, corn, eggs, and nightshades. An elimination diet or food sensitivity testing can help identify problematic foods.
2. **Remove Processed Foods and Refined Sugars:** Ultra-processed foods and added sugars promote inflammation and feed harmful gut bacteria. Replacing these with whole, nutrient-dense foods like vegetables, fruits, nuts, and seeds supports a balanced microbiome.
3. **Minimize Antibiotic Overuse:** While sometimes necessary, antibiotics disrupt the gut microbiome by eliminating both harmful and beneficial bacteria. Work with a healthcare provider to use antibiotics only when essential and support recovery with eating a diet rich in polyphenols, a wide variety of fruits and vegetables, fermented foods and probiotics.
4. **Manage Stress:** Chronic stress negatively impacts gut health by altering gut motility, microbiota composition and increases gut permeability (leaky gut). Techniques like deep breathing, mindfulness, spending quiet time in nature and yoga can help regulate stress and improve digestion.
5. **Remove Harmful Pathogens:** Pathogenic bacteria, yeast overgrowth (such as Candida), and parasitic worms can damage gut health. Symptoms like persistent bloating, diarrhea, or recurrent infections may indicate an infection. Stool testing can help identify these pathogens and guide targeted removal strategies. Disease causing bacteria and yeast can easily grow out of control from a combination or in isolation of consuming sugar, processed foods, preservatives, antibiotic use, environmental toxins, excess alcohol, eating moldy food, nutrient

devoid diet and more.

Natural Remedies for Gut Pathogen Removal

Important: It is wise to undertake gut-cleansing protocols under the guidance of an experienced practitioner. Testing (such as comprehensive microbiome analysis) is essential to identify specific pathogens and determine the most appropriate remedies, dosages, and duration. These interventions are not recommended during pregnancy or breastfeeding and should be avoided - if you have pre-existing health conditions undertaking pathogen removal should be carefully supervised -

Any of these remedies should be started on its own at a low dose, and gradually increase only as tolerated. This approach helps minimize the risk of a Herxheimer reaction (or Herx reaction) - a temporary, inflammatory response that can occur when large numbers of pathogens (bacteria, fungi, parasites) die off and release toxins into the bloodstream. This die-off can temporarily overwhelm the body's detoxification systems, leading to symptoms like nausea, fatigue, headaches, brain fog, joint pain, or flu-like discomfort.

Natural antimicrobials such as oregano oil, berberine, and garlic are commonly used to target harmful microbes and may trigger a Herx reaction. The severity of symptoms often reflects how well your liver, kidneys, lymphatic system, and bowels are eliminating the resulting toxins.

To reduce discomfort during this process:

- Stay well hydrated.
- Support liver function with antioxidants (e.g., milk thistle, NAC).
- Consume dietary fiber to aid toxin elimination.
- Temporarily reduce the dose if symptoms become severe.
- Consider binders such as activated charcoal or bentonite clay to help mop up released toxins (especially mycotoxins).

- Use high-quality probiotics to support microbiome balance and prevent the overgrowth of opportunistic organisms.
- Keep elimination pathways open - if you're constipated, address that before beginning pathogen removal.

While uncomfortable, a Herx reaction can be a sign that the treatment is working and that your body is clearing out harmful microbes - just proceed cautiously and always with professional support.

- **Oregano Oil**: Contains carvacrol and thymol, which combat bacterial and fungal overgrowths. Supports gut healing and reduces inflammation. Use short-term and pair with probiotics to maintain microbial balance.
- **Berberine**: Targets bacterial infections like H. pylori and SIBO. Reduces gut inflammation and helps regulate blood sugar. May interact with medications—consult a healthcare provider before use.
- **Garlic (Allicin)**: Has antibacterial, antifungal, and anti-parasitic properties. Supports immune function and gut microbiome balance. Aged garlic supplements can reduce digestive irritation.
- **Psyllium Husk**: A fiber-rich prebiotic that aids in detoxification and supports beneficial bacteria. Helps eliminate toxins, heavy metals, and metabolic waste. Regulates bowel movements and promotes microbiome diversity. Psyllium can be easily added to water, smoothies, or meals for its gut-cleansing benefits.
- **Coconut Oil**: Contains medium-chain triglycerides (MCTs) and lauric acid, which have antimicrobial, antifungal, and antiviral properties. Supports gut health by reducing harmful bacteria like Candida and promoting healthy digestion. Use extra virgin coconut oil for maximum benefits. These MCTs can help reduce harmful gut bacteria while supporting a balanced microbiome.
- **Apple Cider Vinegar (ACV)**: Contains acetic acid, which has antimicrobial properties that can help balance gut bacteria and inhibit harmful pathogens. Supports digestion by increasing stomach acid production, aiding in the breakdown of food and nutrient absorption. It also supports

bile production, enhancing digestion and detoxification. Opt for raw, unfiltered ACV with the "mother" for the best effects. Enjoy a couple of tablespoons in a large glass of filtered water each morning.

- **Wormwood (Artemisia absinthium):** A powerful anti-parasitic herb traditionally used for intestinal worms, especially roundworms and pinworms. It contains compounds like thujone that disrupt parasite metabolism.
- **Black Walnut Hull (Juglans nigra):** Rich in tannins and juglone, this is a potent remedy often paired with wormwood. It helps eliminate both adult worms and their eggs, particularly effective against tapeworms and ringworms.
- **Clove (Syzygium aromaticum):** High in eugenol, cloves kill parasite eggs and have strong antifungal, antibacterial, and antiparasitic properties. Often used with wormwood and black walnut for a synergistic effect.
- **Papaya Seeds:** Contain enzymes like papain and caricin, which can digest and kill parasites. Studies have shown effectiveness against intestinal worms when combined with honey.
- **Pumpkin Seeds (Cucurbita pepo):** Contain cucurbitacin, a compound that paralyzes worms, especially tapeworms and roundworms, allowing them to be expelled. Best eaten raw and ground.
- **Neem (Azadirachta indica):** Traditional Ayurvedic herb that disrupts parasite reproduction and starves them. Also has antibacterial and blood-purifying properties.
- **Diatomaceous Earth (Food Grade Only):** Particles of earth that can pierce and dehydrate parasites in the gut. Must be taken with plenty of water and only in food-grade form.

Remove Environmental Toxins

Environmental toxins - such as heavy metals, agricultural chemicals, synthetic food additives, and compounds found in personal care products- can accumulate in the body over time. These toxins are known to disrupt the gut microbiome, impair detoxification pathways, contribute to chronic inflammation, and interfere with hormone function. Reducing your exposure is an essential step toward healing and restoring balance.

Minimize Heavy Metal Exposure

Heavy metals like mercury, lead, arsenic, and cadmium are toxic to the gut and nervous system, and may impair mitochondrial function and detoxification.

- Avoid high-mercury fish such as tuna, swordfish, and king mackerel, especially for children and during pregnancy.
- Consider safe removal of amalgam fillings under the supervision of a biological dentist, as these may release mercury vapor.
- Reduce exposure to air pollution, cigarette smoke, and industrial environments where heavy metals may be present in dust and particulates.
- Support natural detoxification with foods rich in sulfur (e.g., garlic, onions, cruciferous vegetables) and binders like chlorella or cilantro, under practitioner guidance.

Reduce Exposure to Agricultural and Household Chemicals

Many synthetic chemicals used in farming and cleaning—such as glyphosate, pesticides, and VOCs (volatile organic compounds)—have been linked to gut dysbiosis, endocrine disruption, and systemic inflammation.

- Choose organic and regenerative foods wherever possible, particularly for high-residue crops like berries, apples, grapes, spinach, and capsicum, which often carry high pesticide loads.
- Organic and regeneratively raised meats and dairy help limit intake of

antibiotics, hormones, and synthetic feed additives that can disrupt your gut and hormonal balance.
- Avoid plastic containers, plastic wrap, and non-stick cookware, which may leach hormone-disrupting chemicals such as BPA, phthalates, and PFAS into your food. Opt for glass, stainless steel, or ceramic alternatives.
- Switch to non-toxic cleaning products, avoiding ingredients like bleach, ammonia, synthetic fragrances, and quaternary ammonium compounds, all of which can irritate the gut and respiratory tract.

Choose Natural Personal Care Products

Daily use of personal care products can contribute significantly to your body's chemical burden, especially when applied to skin, where absorption is direct.

- Common ingredients like parabens, phthalates, sulfates, triclosan, and synthetic fragrances are known endocrine disruptors and possible carcinogens.
- Opt for fragrance-free, certified organic, or low-tox alternatives for items such as body wash, toothpaste, shampoo, deodorant, lotions, and cosmetics.

Be especially mindful during pregnancy or early childhood, when endocrine and neurological systems are more sensitive to disruption.

Step 2: Replace – Restore Digestive Support

Duration: Often concurrent with Step 1

- **Stomach acid support**: betaine HCl or apple cider vinegar (if low stomach acid is determined).
- **Digestive enzymes**: support breakdown and absorption of food, especially helpful if bloating, gas, or undigested food in stool is present.

- **Bile support**: bitter herbs like dandelion root or artichoke for fat digestion if gallbladder sluggishness is suspected.

Step 3: Repair – Healing the Gut Lining

Duration: 4 to 12 weeks+ for mild gut lining damage follow for 4 weeks however for severe cases (IBS, IBD, autoimmune gut conditions) longer than 12 weeks with ongoing maintenance is to be expected.

Once irritants are removed, the next critical step in gut restoration is repairing the gut lining. The gut lining acts as a protective barrier, allowing essential nutrients to be absorbed while keeping harmful substances out of the bloodstream. However, modern diets, stress, and environmental toxins can compromise this delicate lining, leading to a condition called increased intestinal permeability – often referred to as "leaky gut." Factors such as ultra-processed foods, excessive sugar, refined carbohydrates, food additives, alcohol, chronic stress, and medications like antibiotics or non-steroidal anti-inflammatory drugs (NSAIDs) can weaken the intestinal lining over time. Additionally, imbalances in gut bacteria (dysbiosis) and exposure to environmental toxins, including pesticides and heavy metals, can further degrade gut integrity.

When the gut lining becomes damaged, harmful particles such as undigested food proteins, toxins, and bacteria can pass into the bloodstream, triggering widespread inflammation. This can contribute to various health problems, including digestive disorders like bloating, gas, and irritable bowel syndrome (IBS). Beyond digestion, a weakened gut lining has been linked to autoimmune conditions, food sensitivities, skin issues like eczema, and even mental health concerns such as anxiety and depression due to the gut-brain connection.

Why is Gut Repair Essential?

- **Restores Gut Barrier Integrity**: A strong gut lining prevents harmful substances from entering the bloodstream.
- **Enhances Nutrient Absorption**: Proper digestion and assimilation of essential vitamins, minerals, and amino acids rely on a well-functioning gut lining.
- **Reduces Inflammation**: Healing the gut reduces chronic inflammation, improving symptoms of conditions like IBS, gastritis, and autoimmune disorders.
- **Supports Immune Health**: Since 70% of the immune system resides in the gut, a healthy intestinal barrier is crucial for overall immune function.

Key Tools for Gut Lining Repair

1. Nutrient Support: Zinc Carnosine

Zinc carnosine is a compound that protects and repairs the gut lining by forming a protective layer over damaged tissue and promoting healing. Benefits of zinc carnosine include:

- **Repairs & Protects the Gut Lining**: Helps heal damage caused by NSAIDs, infections, and chronic inflammation.
- **Reduces Inflammation**: Beneficial for gastritis, IBD, and leaky gut.
- **Boosts Immune Function**: Zinc enhances immune defense against gut pathogens.
- **Neutralizes Free Radicals**: Reduces oxidative stress that contributes to gut damage.

2. Structural Support: Collagen Peptides

Collagen peptides contain amino acids like glycine and proline, which are essential for maintaining and rebuilding gut integrity. Benefits of collagen peptides and gelatin include:

- **Strengthens the Gut Barrier**: Supports tight junctions in the intestinal wall.
- **Reduces Inflammation**: Helps repair leaky gut and inflammatory conditions.
- **Aids in Digestive Health**: Provides nourishment for gut cells and supports tissue regeneration.

3. Colostrum

Bovine colostrum is the nutrient-rich "first milk" produced by cows in the first 24–72 hours after giving birth. It's packed with growth factors, immunoglobulins, and antimicrobial peptides that support gut, immune, and overall mucosal health. Benefits of Colostrum include:

- **Seals and Heals the Gut Lining:** Contains growth factors like IGF-1 and TGF-β, which help regenerate intestinal cells and tighten the gut barrier.
- **Reduces Inflammation:** Helps calm immune activation in the gut and may reduce symptoms of leaky gut, IBD, and food sensitivities.
- **Supports Immune Function:** Rich in immunoglobulins (especially IgG), which help defend against pathogens and restore immune balance in the gut.
- **Promotes Microbiome Health:** Encourages the growth of beneficial bacteria and creates an environment that discourages pathogens and overgrowth.
- Colostrum is generally well-tolerated, but dairy-sensitive individuals should use caution and opt for low-lactose or third-party-tested forms. It's especially helpful during recovery from infections, antibiotic use, or

postnatal depletion.

4. Gut Microbiome Support: Probiotics

Probiotics (beneficial bacteria) help restore microbial balance, reduce inflammation, enhance the mucosal barrier – all of which are crucial for gut lining repair. To heal the gut lining, the best probiotics to heal the gut barrier are as follows:

Lactobacillus species

- **Lactobacillus rhamnosus GG**: Helps strengthen the gut lining, reduce leaky gut, and modulate the immune system.
- **Lactobacillus reuteri**: Supports mucosal integrity and reduces inflammation.
- **Lactobacillus plantarum**: Aids in healing the intestinal barrier and reducing gut permeability.

Bifidobacterium species

- **Bifidobacterium breve**: Supports short-chain fatty acid (SCFA) production, promoting gut lining repair.
- **Bifidobacterium longum**: Reduces inflammation and helps restore the gut microbiome.
- **Bifidobacterium bifidum**: Enhances mucin production, which protects the gut lining.

Soil-Based Organisms (SBOs)

- **Bacillus coagulans**: Helps reduce gut inflammation and supports tight junction integrity.
- **Bacillus subtilis** – Aids in pathogen control while promoting a balanced microbiome.

Saccharomyces boulardii (Beneficial Yeast): Supports gut lining repair by increasing IgA (an immune-supporting antibody). Reduces inflammation and prevents harmful bacteria from adhering to the gut wall.

Spore-Forming Probiotics: Help survive stomach acid and reach the intestines intact. Support gut resilience and help repair damage from dysbiosis.

5. Anti-Inflammatory Support: Aloe Vera

Aloe vera contains bioactive compounds that reduce gut inflammation and promote healing. Benefits of Aloe Vera:

- **Soothes Digestive Discomfort:** Helps with acid reflux, bloating, and gastritis.
- **Repairs Intestinal Barrier**: Aids in healing leaky gut and ulcerative conditions.
- **Supports Immune Function**: Contains antimicrobial properties to protect against harmful bacteria.

Step 4: Restore — Rebuilding the Microbiome

Duration: 4–8 weeks, depending on your gut microbiome test results.

With the gut lining repaired, the final step is to restore the microbiome — the trillions of bacteria, fungi, and other microorganisms that live in the gut and influence digestion, immunity, hormone balance, and mental health.

This complex internal ecosystem is easily disrupted by antibiotics, processed foods, stress, and illness — leading to symptoms like digestive discomfort, weakened immunity, and mood imbalances. The gut's far-reaching influence has earned it the nickname *"the second brain"* — it produces about 90% of the body's serotonin, a key neurotransmitter for mood regulation.

Restoring microbial balance is essential for long-term health and vitality. Fortunately, there are science-backed tools to support this process, including **probiotics, prebiotics,** and **gut-friendly lifestyle therapies**.

1. Probiotics: Replenishing Beneficial Bacteria

Probiotics are live microorganisms that help repopulate beneficial gut bacteria, outcompete harmful microbes, and support digestion, immune function, and emotional well-being.

Sources of Probiotics:

- *Fermented foods*: yogurt, kefir, sauerkraut, kimchi, miso, tempeh, kombucha
- *Supplements*: Opt for high-quality, multi-strain formulas (aim for at least 10 billion CFUs and 10+ strains), ideally selected based on microbiome test results

Key Strains & Benefits:

- *Lactobacillus rhamnosus*: Strengthens the gut lining and reduces diarrhea
- *Bifidobacterium longum*: Modulates inflammation and supports mood
- *Saccharomyces boulardii*: A beneficial yeast that protects against antibiotic-related diarrhea and enhances gut resilience

How Probiotics Help:

- Rebalance the gut after illness, antibiotics, or poor diet
- Improve digestion by aiding in the breakdown of carbohydrates, proteins, and fats
- Boost immune defenses by enhancing gut barrier function
- Reduce inflammation and help manage conditions like IBS and leaky gut

Signs You May Benefit from Probiotics:

- Bloating, gas, or constipation
- Recurrent infections (gut, urinary tract, sinus)
- Skin issues (acne, eczema, rosacea)
- IBS or inflammatory bowel symptoms
- Anxiety or low mood

Potential Side Effects & Tips:

- *Temporary bloating/gas*: Start with a low dose and increase gradually
- *Caution for immunocompromised individuals*: Consult your healthcare provider before use

2. Prebiotics: Nourishing Your Good Bacteria

Prebiotics are non-digestible fibers that serve as food for your beneficial gut bacteria, helping them grow and thrive.

Types & Food Sources:

- *Inulin & FOS*: Onions, garlic, leeks, asparagus, bananas
- *GOS*: Dairy products, legumes
- *Resistant starch*: Cooked and cooled potatoes, green bananas, oats, whole grains

How They Work:

Prebiotics selectively feed bacteria like *Bifidobacteria* and *Lactobacilli*, enhancing production of **short-chain fatty acids** (SCFAs) like butyrate, which support gut lining integrity, reduce inflammation, and improve mineral absorption (e.g., calcium, magnesium, iron).

Benefits of Prebiotics:

- Improve bowel regularity and reduce bloating
- Enhance immune response and protection against harmful microbes
- Support mood and cognition via SCFA production

- Help manage inflammatory conditions like IBS and metabolic syndrome

Signs You May Need Prebiotics:

- Chronic bloating or irregular bowel movements
- Frequent infections or low immunity
- Poor mineral absorption or low bone density
- Food cravings or blood sugar instability

Potential Side Effects & Tips:

- *Gas and bloating*: Common when increasing fiber — introduce slowly
- *Cramps or loose stools*: Avoid overconsumption; 5–10g daily is ideal
- *Hydration is essential*: Drink plenty of water to aid fiber digestion

3. Lifestyle Strategies to Support a Healthy Microbiome

In addition to dietary approaches, your daily habits can significantly influence your gut health.

Eat a Diverse, Plant-Rich Diet

- Aim for 30+ different plant foods per week to boost microbial diversity
- Include polyphenol-rich foods (berries, green tea, dark chocolate, olive oil) that feed good bacteria

Prioritize Quality Sleep

- Disrupted circadian rhythms negatively affect the gut microbiome
- Aim for 7–9 hours of restful sleep each night

Stay Physically Active

- Regular movement enhances microbiome diversity and improves gut

motility
- Even gentle activity like walking can support microbial balance

16

Enhancing Your Energy

It's normal to feel tired occasionally, but if you find yourself constantly exhausted, collapsing by the end of the day and still not feeling rested despite a full night's sleep, there may be an underlying issue that needs attention.

If you find yourself reaching for a second cup of coffee, energy drink or sugary treats just to get through the day, it is important to remember that while these quick fixes might offer a temporary lift, they often lead to crashes that leave you feeling more exhausted. In such cases, it's tempting to reach for a quick fix like another cup of coffee or a sugary treat to give you another burst of energy. However, when you're already feeling depleted, these short-term solutions can worsen your fatigue in the long run.

Although I am a fan of good quality organic coffee, consuming too much coffee can be problematic for your energy levels, as it can overstimulate your adrenal glands and disrupt your cortisol levels, which are essential for managing stress and regulating sleep. High caffeine intake may lead to a temporary energy spike, but it ultimately contributes to adrenal fatigue and can interfere with the quality of your sleep. This cyclical pattern of energy crashes and poor sleep can exacerbate feelings of fatigue over time.

Similarly, consuming excess sugar may give you an immediate energy surge, but it can have detrimental effects on your energy levels in the long term. When you eat sugary foods, your blood sugar levels spike rapidly, followed by a sharp crash that leaves you feeling even more tired and sluggish. Repeated spikes and crashes can disrupt your body's energy regulation and lead to chronic fatigue.

Furthermore, a diet high in sugar can negatively impact your gut health. Sugar feeds harmful bacteria in the gut, which can create an imbalance in the microbiome. This imbalance is linked to various health issues, including fatigue, as it affects nutrient absorption, hormone production, and overall energy regulation.

In summary, while sugar and caffeine may offer a temporary energy boost, their long-term impact on the body – particularly on adrenal function, sleep quality, and gut health – can significantly hinder your ability to maintain consistent energy levels

Natural Energy Boosters

Fatigue is often linked to impaired energy production at the cellular level. Mitochondria, the energy-producing structures within cells, are essential for maintaining normal cell function. When mitochondria are damaged, it can be a primary factor contributing to feelings of fatigue. Such damage is typically caused by poor dietary habits and lifestyle choices, which promote the formation of free radicals. Free radicals are unstable molecules that can damage cells, mitochondria, and DNA. When mitochondrial function is compromised, energy production decreases, leading to fatigue. Improving mitochondrial health is therefore crucial for increasing energy levels. Antioxidants help neutralize free radicals, protecting the body from cellular damage and supporting energy production.

Before you reach for another coffee, energy drink or sugar hit, consider these natural supplements to fuel your day. Science supports a range of natural supplements that can enhance your energy levels sustainably and safely. However, while each option has unique benefits, you should consult with a healthcare provider before starting any new supplement regimen, especially if you have underlying health conditions, are pregnant or breastfeeding or are taking medications.

Maintain Blood Sugar Balance for Energy

Before reaching for the supplements, first get into habits that will help you maintain stable blood sugar levels – this is crucial for consistent energy and mood stability. Fluctuations in blood sugar can lead to feelings of fatigue, irritability, and low energy. To support blood sugar balance:

1. **Eat Regularly:** Have regular meals and snacks to keep blood sugar levels steady.
2. **Choose Low Glycemic Index Foods**: Opt for foods that release energy slowly, such as whole grains, legumes, and vegetables.
3. **Incorporate Protein and Healthy Fats:** Adding protein and healthy fats to meals can help slow the absorption of carbohydrates and maintain stable blood sugar levels.

Magnesium: The Silent Energy Hero

Magnesium plays a starring role in over 300 biochemical reactions in your body, many of which involve energy production. A deficiency in magnesium can leave you feeling sluggish, cranky, and even prone to muscle cramps. Research shows that magnesium deficiency is surprisingly common, affecting up to 50% of people in developed countries. Soil depletion and processed foods are major culprits. When replenished, magnesium has been shown to improve physical performance and reduce fatigue, particularly in older adults.

Try This: Incorporate magnesium-rich foods like almonds, spinach, and dark chocolate into your diet or consider a high-quality supplement.

Iron: Oxygen's Best Friend

Iron is essential for producing haemoglobin, the protein in red blood cells that carries oxygen to your tissues. Low iron levels can cause anemia, making you feel perpetually tired and weak. Iron deficiency is the most widespread nutrient deficiency in the world, affecting over 2 billion people. A clinical update revealed that treating iron deficiency anemia can significantly improve energy, focus, and even mood.

Try This: Boost your iron intake with foods like red meat, lentils, and fortified cereals. Pair these with vitamin C-rich foods to enhance absorption.

Coenzyme Q10: The Cellular Powerhouse

Coenzyme Q10, or CoQ10, is a naturally occurring compound that helps your cells produce energy. This antioxidant also protects your body from oxidative stress, a common energy drainer. As we age, our natural CoQ10 levels drop, and certain medications, like cholesterol-lowering statins, further deplete this vital compound. Studies have shown that CoQ10 supplementation can alleviate fatigue and improve energy, particularly in individuals with chronic fatigue syndrome.

Try This: Consider a daily CoQ10 supplement, especially if you're over 40 or on statins.

Rhodiola Rosea: The Stress Buster

Feeling drained from stress? Rhodiola Rosea, a powerful adaptogenic herb, may be the answer. Adaptogens help balance your body's stress response, reducing the physical and mental toll of life's demands. Traditionally used in Siberia to combat harsh conditions, Rhodiola has been shown to improve mental focus and reduce fatigue, particularly in high-stress environments.

Try This: Look for a standardized Rhodiola Rosea supplement or brew it as tea for a daily stress-relieving ritual.

Vitamin B12: Energy's Best Ally

Vitamin B12 is crucial for red blood cell production, DNA synthesis, and nerve health. A deficiency can lead to fatigue, brain fog, and even neurological issues. Unlike other vitamins, B12 is primarily found in animal products, putting vegans and vegetarians at a higher risk for deficiency. Studies confirm that B12 supplementation can significantly enhance energy and cognitive function in deficient individuals.

Try This: Include more B12-rich foods like eggs, salmon, and dairy in your diet. For those on plant-based diets, a daily B12 supplement is essential.

Other B Vitamins: A Team of Energy Boosters

Vitamin B1 (thiamine), B2 (riboflavin), B3 (niacin), B5 (pantothenic acid), B6 (pyridoxine), B7 (biotin), B9 (folate), and B12 all play key roles in converting the food you eat into energy. They support mitochondrial function and contribute to overall vitality. Deficiencies in B vitamins can lead to fatigue, poor concentration, and mood imbalances. For example, vitamin B6 is involved in the production of serotonin and dopamine, neurotransmitters that influence mood and energy levels. Research has shown that B-complex vitamins can help combat fatigue, particularly in individuals with a deficiency.

Try This: Consider a B-complex supplement if you're feeling drained, ensure that the b-vitamins are in methylated or active form for optimal results. Plus boost your intake with foods like leafy greens and legumes.

Iodine: The Thyroid Energizer

Iodine is essential for thyroid function, which regulates metabolism and energy production. Low iodine levels can impair thyroid hormone production, leading to fatigue, weight gain, and brain fog. Iodine deficiency is one of the most common nutritional deficiencies worldwide, impacting energy levels by disrupting thyroid function. Adequate iodine intake is crucial for maintaining normal thyroid hormone levels, which directly affect energy, metabolism, and mental clarity.

Try This: Include iodine-rich foods like seaweed and iodized salt in your diet to support your thyroid and keep energy levels stable.

Ashwagandha: The Ancient Energy Booster

Ashwagandha, often referred to as "Indian ginseng," is a cornerstone of Ayurvedic medicine. This adaptogen helps reduce stress and improve endurance by enhancing oxygen utilization. Modern studies back up its traditional use, showing that Ashwagandha improves energy levels, reduces stress, and even boosts physical performance.

Try This: Add ashwagandha powder to smoothies or opt for a supplement for consistent benefits.

Creatine: Not Just for Athletes

Creatine is well-known in the fitness world for its ability to enhance muscle strength and performance. But did you know it can also boost energy for non-athletes? Creatine helps regenerate ATP, the energy currency of your cells. Research shows it improves mental clarity and physical endurance, even in people who aren't hitting the gym.

Try This: Take a daily creatine supplement and enjoy increased energy for both body and mind.

Ginseng: The Ancient Root of Vitality

Ginseng, especially Panax ginseng, has long been prized for its energizing properties. This adaptogen enhances cellular energy production and helps regulate blood sugar levels. Ginseng has been shown to reduce fatigue and improve cognitive function during mentally demanding tasks. It's also celebrated for its anti-aging benefits.

Try This: Sip on ginseng tea or take a supplement to combat daily fatigue.

17

Building a Robust Immune System

The immune system is the body's natural defense mechanism against harmful invaders such as bacteria, viruses, and fungi. In a mother's daily life, supporting her immune system is crucial for maintaining not only her health but also her ability to care for her family.

Supporting your immune health is essential for thriving in the demanding role of motherhood. The immune system is a complex, multifaceted network, and understanding how to support it through diet, lifestyle choices, and supplements can help you feel more resilient and ready to take on the challenges of parenthood.

As children begin daycare or school, parent – especially mothers – may notice an increase in the frequency of illnesses, colds, and flu outbreaks. While these illnesses are a natural part of a child's development and exposure to germs, mothers often find themselves at the frontline of managing not only their own health but also their families.

Research shows that immune health is closely tied to a variety of factors, including nutrition, lifestyle choices, environmental influences and gut health. Studies show that approximately 70-80% of the immune system is located in the gut so what you put inside your gut is critical to immune health.

A robust immune system is essential for preventing infections and promoting overall wellness for both mothers and their children. This chapter explores how mothers can support their immune systems and those of their families through nutrition, lifestyle adjustments, and understanding the role of gut health and other immune system factors.

How a Healthy Gut Strengthens Your Immune System

The microbiome, the trillions of microorganisms living in the digestive tract, plays a crucial role in immune health. Research has shown that a healthy gut microbiome is essential for immune function, as it helps synthesize vitamins, absorb nutrients, and protect against harmful pathogens. However, factors such as poor diet, stress, and overuse of antibiotics can disrupt the balance of beneficial bacteria in the gut, leading to weakened immunity.

Strong Stomach Acid Fights Pathogens

Low stomach acid can have a detrimental effect on how robust your immune health is. A properly acidic stomach (with a pH level of 1-2) helps to kill harmful bacteria and pathogens, preventing them from setting up shop and growing in your body. When stomach acid levels are too low, it can allow harmful bacteria to thrive in the gut, contributing to infections and digestive issues. Proton pump inhibitors (PPIs), commonly prescribed for acid reflux, can reduce stomach acid levels and disrupt the gut microbiome, leading to increased vulnerability to infections.

To support healthy stomach acid levels, it is important to chew food thoroughly to increase the body's ability to release digestive enzymes. Consuming fermented foods, bitter foods, using digestive enzymes, and reducing sugar intake can also help. Organic apple cider vinegar, diluted in water, is also an effective natural remedy to improve stomach acidity and support digestion.

Antibiotics Disrupt Your Defenses

Antibiotics have saved millions of lives, but their overuse can have long-term negative effects on gut health and immunity. Antibiotics can wipe out both harmful and beneficial bacteria, disrupting the microbiome and reducing the body's ability to fight infections. This disruption can lead to a weakened immune system and increased susceptibility to infections.

Research shows that a healthy microbiome is essential for immune function, with 70-80% of immune cells located in the gut. It is especially important to avoid unnecessary antibiotics in young children, as their immune systems and microbiomes are still developing.

Immune-Boosting Foods and Functional Ingredients

Our immune system is our body's frontline defense, and maintaining its strength can be greatly supported by the foods we eat. A balanced diet rich in vitamins, minerals, antioxidants, and other beneficial compounds not only fuels our everyday activities but also reinforces our immune response. This guide explores both classic immune-supportive foods and functional ingredients – like apple cider vinegar and bone broth – that can be integrated into your diet for added benefits.

Immune-Supportive Foods: The Basics

Fruits and Vegetables: Fruits and vegetables provide essential vitamins, minerals, and antioxidants that help protect immune cells from oxidative damage. Here are some key examples:

- **Citrus Fruits (Oranges, Lemons, Limes, Grapefruits):** High in vitamin C, which is known to stimulate the production of white blood cells and enhance immune function.
- **Berries (Blueberries, Strawberries, Blackberries, Raspberries):** Packed with antioxidants and vitamins to fight inflammation and oxidative stress.
- **Leafy Greens (Spinach, Kale, Swiss Chard):** Provide vitamins A, C, and E, along with fiber and antioxidants, supporting overall immune health.

- **Cruciferous Vegetables (Broccoli, Brussels Sprouts, Cauliflower):** Rich in vitamins, minerals, and fiber, with compounds that may help reduce inflammation and support detoxification.

Proteins: Proteins are vital for the repair and regeneration of body tissues, including those that form the immune system. High-quality proteins also supply essential nutrients such as zinc.

- **Grass Fed, Free Range Meats and Wild Caught Fish (Beef, Chicken, Turkey, Salmon, Sardines, Trout):** Provide high-quality protein and nutrients like zinc and omega-3 fatty acids, which support immune cell development, repair and reduce inflammation.
- **Legumes (Beans, Lentils, Chickpeas):** Excellent sources of plant-based protein, fiber, and micronutrients.
- **Nuts and Seeds (Almonds, Sunflower Seeds, Walnuts):** Rich in vitamin E and healthy fats, crucial for maintaining cell membranes and moderating inflammation

Healthy Fats: Incorporating healthy fats is important for reducing inflammation and ensuring the proper absorption of fat-soluble vitamins.

- **Omega-3 Rich Foods (Salmon, Sardines, Walnuts):** These fats help maintain cell membrane integrity and reduce inflammation.
- **Olive Oil and Avocado:** Contain monounsaturated fats with anti-inflammatory properties.

Fermented Foods: Fermented foods are renowned for their probiotics, which support gut health—a key factor in overall immune function. Probiotic rich foods (yogurt, kefir, sauerkraut, kimchi) promote a healthy gut microbiome, enhancing digestion and immune regulation.

Spices and Herbs: Certain spices and herbs are known for their potent anti-inflammatory and antioxidant properties. Garlic, ginger, turmeric, oregano, rosemary can help reduce inflammation and combat infections through their antimicrobial and antioxidant effects.

Apple Cider Vinegar (ACV): Apple Cider Vinegar (ACV) offers several potential health benefits. Its antimicrobial properties may help reduce harmful bacteria in the digestive tract, supporting overall gut health. Additionally, ACV can aid digestion by enhancing stomach acid production and assisting in the breakdown of food. Some studies also suggest that ACV may contribute to blood sugar regulation, helping to moderate blood sugar levels. To use ACV effectively, dilute 1–2 tablespoons in a glass of water before meals or incorporate it into salad dressings for added flavor and health benefits.

Bone Broth: Bone broth is a nutrient-rich food with several potential health benefits. It is rich in collagen and gelatin, which help support gut integrity, joint health, and tissue repair. Additionally, it contains amino acids like glycine and proline, which play a role in antibody production and inflammation regulation. Bone broth also provides essential minerals such as calcium, magnesium, and phosphorus, contributing to overall well-being. To incorporate bone broth into your diet, enjoy it as a warm beverage or use it as a base for soups and stews, enhancing both flavor and nutritional value.

Key Nutrients to Boost Immune Health

Nutrition plays a pivotal role in maintaining a strong immune system. Nutrients such as vitamin C, vitamin D, zinc, and probiotics have all been shown to support immune function and reduce the duration and severity of illnesses. Research indicates that a balanced diet rich in these nutrients can significantly reduce the likelihood of infections and contribute to a faster recovery when illness does strike.

Vitamin C: Vitamin C is a well-known immune booster. It helps stimulate the production of white blood cells, which are essential for fighting infections. Citrus fruits, strawberries, kiwi, bell peppers, and broccoli are all excellent sources of vitamin C. Consuming these foods regularly can help keep the immune system functioning optimally.

Vitamin D: Vitamin D, often called the "sunshine vitamin," is essential for immune regulation. Studies have shown that low levels of vitamin D are associated with an increased risk of infections, including respiratory illnesses. Vitamin D is found in fatty fish such as salmon and tuna, egg yolks, and fortified foods like milk and cereals.

Zinc: Zinc is vital for the development and function of immune cells. A deficiency in zinc can impair immune function, making the body more susceptible to infections. Good sources of zinc include oysters, beef, chicken, beans, nuts, and whole grains. Including zinc-rich foods in your diet can help support immune function and maintain overall health.

Probiotics: The gut microbiome plays a major role in the immune system. Probiotics, or beneficial bacteria, are essential for maintaining gut health. Yogurt, fermented foods like kimchi and sauerkraut, and probiotic supplements can help enhance the diversity of gut bacteria, supporting the immune system's ability to fight off infections.

Immune-Boosting Meal Plan

This sample day blends immune-supportive nutrients, gut-healing ingredients, and anti-inflammatory whole foods to strengthen your natural defenses.

Morning

Warm Lemon Water + Apple Cider Vinegar
Start your day with a glass of warm filtered water, fresh lemon juice, and 1 tsp to 1 tbsp of raw, unfiltered apple cider vinegar. This supports healthy stomach acid and digestion.

Organic Green Tea
Packed with polyphenols and antioxidants like EGCG, green tea helps combat oxidative stress and supports a healthy gut microbiome.

Optional Boost: Add a pinch of turmeric and black pepper to your tea for anti-inflammatory benefits.

Breakfast

Greek Yogurt Parfait with Berry Compote and Seeds

- Full-fat Greek yogurt (probiotic-rich)
- Mixed berries (vitamin C, antioxidants, polyphenols)
- Chia or flaxseeds (fiber + omega-3s)
- Walnuts (vitamin E and anti-inflammatory fats)
- Optional: drizzle of raw honey or sprinkle of cinnamon

Upgrade Tip: Add a spoonful of **prebiotic-rich** stewed apple or cooked pear for gut-healing pectin.

Mid-Morning Snack

Fruit + Nut Combo

- Sliced apple or kiwi (vitamin C, fiber, enzymes)
- Handful of activated almonds or sunflower seeds (vitamin E, zinc,

magnesium)

Alternative: A boiled egg for protein and selenium.

Lunch

Rainbow Chicken Salad Bowl

- Mixed leafy greens: spinach, kale, rocket (vitamins A, C, K)
- Shredded purple cabbage or red onion (sulfur-rich + prebiotic)
- Cherry tomatoes, cucumber, grated carrot (fiber + hydration)
- Sliced avocado (healthy fats, glutathione support)
- Grilled chicken or tempeh (protein, zinc, B12)
- Fermented vegetables: sauerkraut or kimchi (probiotics)

Dressing: Extra virgin olive oil, lemon juice, Dijon mustard, turmeric, and black pepper.

Afternoon Snack

Veggie Sticks with Hummus + Bone Broth

- Raw carrots, bell pepper, and celery (prebiotic fiber, vitamin A)
- Hummus (fiber + plant-based protein)
- Cup of warm **bone broth** with added ginger or turmeric (collagen, gut lining support, anti-inflammatory)

Optional Add-on: A Brazil nut (for selenium) or a few olives (polyphenols).

Dinner

- **Lemon Herb Salmon, Quinoa, and Broccoli Plate**
- **Wild salmon**: rich in omega-3s and vitamin D
- **Quinoa**: fiber-rich complete protein
- **Steamed broccoli + garlic**: vitamin C, sulforaphane, prebiotics
- **Brussels sprouts roasted with ghee or EVOO**: support detox and immune defense
- **Herbs**: rosemary, thyme, parsley (antioxidants and antimicrobial compounds)

Optional Side: Small bowl of miso soup (probiotics + trace minerals)

Evening Wind-Down

Herbal Tea

Relax with tulsi (holy basil), lemon balm, or reishi-infused herbal tea to support immune modulation, sleep, and stress reduction.

Optional Snack:

- Small glass of **kefir** or probiotic yogurt
- Add a pinch of cinnamon or cardamom for antimicrobial and blood sugar support

Final Notes

For maximum immune support, your daily plate should include:

- **Colorful plant variety** – for fiber, polyphenols, and antioxidants
- **Fermented & prebiotic foods** – nourish a balanced gut
- **Clean proteins** – to build immune cells and repair tissue

- **Healthy fats** – reduce inflammation and support fat-soluble nutrient absorption
- **Sunshine + D3-rich foods** – for vitamin D
- **Functional extras** – such as ACV, turmeric, bone broth and adaptogens

18

What's on Your Plate? Why Organic Matters

Just a few generations ago, our grandparents ate what would now be considered mostly organic by today's standards — food grown without synthetic pesticides, hormones, or genetically modified ingredients. Fast-forward to today, and modern agricultural practices have dramatically increased the use of chemical sprays, preservatives, and additives, many of which have been linked to health issues, especially for women in their reproductive and caregiving years.

Choosing organic and regeneratively grown food isn't about perfection — it's about reducing your body's daily burden. Organic farming avoids synthetic fertilizers, pesticides, and genetically modified organisms (GMOs), meaning fewer hormone-disrupting chemicals end up in your body. Regenerative farming goes a step further, actively improving soil health and increasing the nutrient density of the food you eat — making it an investment in your long-term wellness.

Research shows that women who eat organic regularly have lower levels of pesticide residues in their bodies. This is particularly important because many of these chemicals act as endocrine disruptors, mimicking or interfering with your natural hormones. Over time, this can contribute to fatigue, thyroid imbalances, PMS, irregular cycles, fertility struggles, and even hormone-driven cancers.

Organic foods also tend to be richer in antioxidants, vitamins, and minerals — the building blocks your body needs to recover from stress, support your immune system, and maintain radiant skin, stable energy, and a clear mind. Organic dairy and grass-fed meat products often contain higher levels of omega-3 fatty acids and fewer inflammatory compounds, supporting brain and hormone health.

Beyond the personal health benefits, choosing organic and regenerative supports a safer food system for everyone. These practices reduce harmful chemical runoff, protect pollinators, and rebuild healthy soil — all of which contribute to a more resilient future for the next generation.

How to Incorporate More Organic Foods Affordably

The benefits of eating organic foods are widely acknowledged, especially given their potential to reduce exposure to pesticide residues and hormone-disrupting chemicals, while offering nutrient-dense options that support long-term health. However, organic foods often come with a higher price tag, making them challenging for those on a budget. Despite this barrier, there are ways to access organic and lower-pesticide foods without breaking the bank. Here are effective strategies for purchasing organic foods affordably:

1. Prioritize the "Dirty Dozen" and "Clean Fifteen"

The Environmental Working Group (EWG) publishes annual lists of the "Dirty Dozen" and "Clean Fifteen," which identify fruits and vegetables with the highest and lowest pesticide residues, respectively (EWG, 2023). For those on a budget, this guide is invaluable in prioritizing which items to buy organic. Produce like strawberries, spinach, kale, nectarines, apples, grapes, peaches, cherries, pears, tomatoes, celery, and potatoes – frequent members of the "Dirty Dozen – are worth buying organic due to their higher pesticide residue levels. Meanwhile, foods like avocados, pineapples, and onions tend to have low pesticide residues and can be bought conventionally with less concern for pesticide exposure.

2. Shop at Farmers' Markets and Local Farms

Farmers' markets often provide a direct link to local, organic, or naturally grown produce, frequently at a lower cost than supermarkets. Some local farmers may use organic methods without official certification due to the high cost of certification. Asking about their farming practices can help determine if their produce aligns with your health goals. Many markets offer discounts near closing times, enabling shoppers to purchase high-quality, pesticide-free produce at reduced prices.

3. Buy in Bulk and Store Wisely

Certain organic foods can be more affordable when bought in bulk. Staples like grains, nuts, seeds, and legumes, which are often grown without heavy pesticide use, tend to be less costly per unit when purchased in larger quantities. Buying items in bulk from warehouse stores or online retailers can help stretch the budget. Additionally, storing bulk items properly can extend their shelf life, allowing for cost savings over time.

4. Consider Frozen Organic Produce

Frozen fruits and vegetables are generally less expensive than their fresh counterparts and are picked at peak ripeness, preserving their nutrient content. Many frozen organic options can be found at lower prices, especially in bulk quantities, providing a cost-effective way to enjoy organic produce year-round. Frozen items also help prevent food waste, as they can be stored longer and used as needed, ultimately saving money.

5. Shop Seasonally and Choose Store Brands

Organic foods are typically less expensive when they're in season due to lower transportation costs and higher availability. Planning meals around what's in season can reduce costs while ensuring fresher, nutrient-rich produce. Many grocery stores also offer their own organic store brands, which are often significantly less expensive than well-known organic brands.

Store-brand organics meet the same USDA Organic certification standards, making them a great choice for budget-conscious shoppers.

6. Grow Your Own Organic Food

For those with the time, space, and interest, growing food at home can be one of the most affordable ways to access organic produce. A small backyard garden, container gardening, or even indoor herbs can provide fresh, pesticide-free food throughout the growing season. Crops like tomatoes, lettuce, and herbs are relatively easy to grow, and starting with seeds rather than seedlings can further reduce costs. Gardening also has additional mental and physical health benefits, making it a rewarding practice overall.

7. Use Food Co-ops and Community-Supported Agriculture (CSA)

Many communities offer food cooperatives and CSA programs, which allow members to share in a farm's produce for a fraction of typical grocery store prices. In a CSA, members pay a subscription fee to receive a weekly or monthly box of seasonal produce, often including organically grown items. While the up-front cost can be higher, the cost per unit is generally lower over the long term, and the produce is often fresher and pesticide-free. Food co-ops also offer bulk discounts and member deals that help reduce costs for organic foods.

8. Prioritize Affordable Organic Animal Products and Plant-Based Proteins

Organic meat and dairy can be expensive due to the higher costs of organic farming. To keep costs down while maintaining quality nutrition, try incorporating more plant-based protein sources like beans, lentils, and quinoa, which are often more affordable than organic meats.

When purchasing animal products:

- Buy in bulk and opt for cheaper cuts like mince or those suitable for slow cooking.
- Choose roasts over steaks—buying a whole roast and slicing it into steaks

yourself can save dollars per pound or kilo.
- Prioritize organic or pastured eggs and dairy, which offer higher omega-3 content and fewer contaminants, providing health benefits without the high cost of going fully organic with all meats.

19

Reducing Harmful Chemicals - Safer Personal Care, Cleaning and Food

Motherhood can bring a heightened awareness of what truly matters — not just in how we live, but in what we're surrounded by. From the lotions we smooth on our skin to the food we place on the table, we're exposed to hundreds of synthetic chemicals each day — many of which were never tested for long-term safety. And while modern life offers convenience, it's come with a cost: invisible toxins now linger in our homes, our diets and our daily routines.

Today, over 350,000 registered chemicals and chemical mixtures are approved for use globally and many of these have minimal testing and regulation. Studies show the average person is exposed to more than 160 chemicals daily from personal care products alone, not to mention the toxins found in cleaning products, plastic packaging, and ultra-processed food. For mothers juggling the demands of modern life, these exposures may seem small — but over time, they accumulate, influencing everything from hormone balance and energy levels to immune health, fertility, and even the way we age.

Certain chemicals — like phthalates, parabens, PFAS, and synthetic fragrances — are known endocrine disruptors, meaning they can interfere with natural hormone signaling. Others can affect respiratory health, gut integrity, skin sensitivity, or even increase cancer risk. The good news is: once you know where these chemicals hide, you can begin to avoid them — not perfectly, but intentionally.

This chapter provides practical guidance on:

- The top chemicals to eliminate or reduce from your home and body
- How to transition to safer personal care and cleaning products
- Simple food swaps to lower dietary chemical exposure
- Everyday habit shifts that protect your long-term vitality

The goal is not perfection — it's empowerment. Because every product you swap and every cleaner you replace with a safer option is a small act of care — for your hormones, your energy, your home, and your future.

The Top Toxins to Eliminate

These are the most important chemicals to avoid in your home, food, and personal care. Many are hormone disruptors, carcinogens, or linked to fertility issues and immune dysfunction—especially concerning for women and developing children.

PFAS ("Forever Chemicals")

- **Where:** Non-stick cookware, microwave popcorn bags, fast food wrappers, stain-resistant fabrics, artificial grass
- **Why Avoid:** These long-lasting chemicals build up in the body. Linked to hormone disruption, lower immunity, infertility, and even found in umbilical cord blood.
- **Tip:** Swap non-stick pans for stainless steel or cast iron. Avoid grease-proof food packaging.

Heavy Metals (Lead, Mercury, Cadmium, Arsenic)

- **Where:** Predatory fish (tuna, swordfish), old paint, tap water (pipes), industrial pollution
- **Why Avoid:** Accumulate in the body and affect fertility, brain development, and immune function.
- **Tip:** Choose smaller fish (sardines, salmon), use water filters, test older homes for lead.

Parabens

- **Where:** Lotions, shampoos, makeup, deodorants
- **Why Avoid:** Mimic estrogen and may disrupt hormone balance. Linked to early puberty and hormone-sensitive cancers.
- **Tip:** Look for "paraben-free" on personal care labels.

Phthalates

- **Where:** Fragrances (in lotions, cleaning products, perfumes), soft plastics, air fresheners
- **Why Avoid:** Interfere with hormone production, fertility, fetal development.
- **Tip:** Avoid scented products unless labeled phthalate-free or naturally fragranced with essential oils.

Formaldehyde

- **Where:** Nail polish, hair treatments, cleaning products, furniture glues
- **Why Avoid:** Known carcinogen. Triggers respiratory issues and skin irritation.
- **Tip:** Choose "formaldehyde-free" products and ventilate when using new furniture or building materials.

Triclosan

- **Where:** Antibacterial soaps, toothpaste, some deodorants
- **Why Avoid:** Disrupts thyroid hormones, may contribute to antibiotic resistance.
- **Tip:** Skip "antibacterial" labels—plain soap and water is just as effective.

Fragrance / Parfum

- **Where:** Anything scented: perfumes, candles, baby wipes, personal care
- **Why Avoid:** Can contain dozens of hidden chemicals including hormone disruptors and allergens.
- **Tip:** Choose fragrance-free or essential oil–scented products. Be cautious with products marketed as "natural."

Chlorine Bleach & Ammonia

- **Where:** Cleaning sprays, toilet bowl cleaners, mold removers
- **Why Avoid:** Can irritate lungs and skin, especially in poorly ventilated areas.
- **Tip:** Switch to natural cleaners like vinegar, baking soda, or castile soap.

How to Reduce Chemicals in Your Diet

Food is one of the biggest daily sources of chemical exposure - but it's also where you have the most control. Here's how to make meaningful swaps without overwhelm:

Prioritize Organic Where It Matters Most

Why: Conventional produce is often sprayed with hormone-disrupting pesticides.
What to Do:

- Use the *Environmental Working Group's Dirty Dozen* list to choose which produce to always buy organic (strawberries, spinach, apples, kale and other leafy greens and stone fruits usually always make this list each year).
- When organic isn't accessible, wash produce thoroughly and peel where possible.

Ditch Ultra-Processed Foods

Why: Packaged foods are loaded with preservatives, artificial colors, flavor enhancers, and emulsifiers that may affect hormones, metabolism, and gut health.
What to Do:

- Cook from scratch when possible.
- Choose products with short, recognizable ingredient lists.
- Avoid "flavored," "diet," and "shelf-stable" snacks that last unnaturally long.

Avoid Artificial Sweeteners & Colors

Why: Linked to gut dysbiosis, metabolic issues, and behavioral concerns.
What to Do:

- Skip aspartame, sucralose, saccharin, and colors like Red 40 and Yellow 5.
- Use raw honey, maple syrup, or stevia in moderation.

- Choose naturally colorful foods (like berries) over dyed treats.

Reduce Plastic Contact with Food

Why: Plastics can leach endocrine-disrupting chemicals (like BPA, BPS, and phthalates), especially when heated.
What to Do:

- Store leftovers in glass or stainless steel containers.
- Avoid microwaving in plastic.
- Choose fresh or frozen food over canned (lined cans may contain BPA).

Watch for Sneaky Additives

What to Limit or Avoid:

- **"Natural flavors"** – can include synthetic solvents and preservatives.
- **"Fat-free" or "sugar-free" products** – often contain additives to mimic texture or taste.
- **Emulsifiers** (like polysorbates and carrageenan) – can alter gut bacteria.

Support Detox with Whole Foods

Why: A healthy gut and liver help your body remove toxins naturally.
What to Do:

- Eat plenty of fiber (vegetables, seeds, lentils) to support bowel regularity.
- Drink filtered water throughout the day.
- Include detox-supportive foods like leafy greens, cruciferous veggies, garlic, lemon, and fermented foods (e.g. sauerkraut, kefir).

Look for Trusted Certifications

Why: Labels help you make informed choices quickly.
What to Look For:

- USDA Organic
- Australian Certified Organic (ACO)
- Non-GMO Project Verified
- Glyphosate Residue Free
- Read the full ingredient list even on "natural" products - greenwashing is common.

Reducing Chemical Exposure in Personal Care & Cleaning Products

Many everyday products marketed as "clean" or "gentle" still contain synthetic chemicals that can irritate the skin, disrupt hormones, or affect long-term health. Here's how to simplify your routines and reduce your toxic load.

Simplify Your Personal Care Routine

Why: The average woman uses 12 personal care products daily, exposing herself to over 160 chemicals - many untested for safety.
What to Do:

- **Go fragrance-free** or choose **essential oil-scented** products (avoid "parfum" or "fragrance" unless specified as natural).
- Swap conventional moisturizers and cleansers for **plant-based products** made with aloe, shea butter, coconut oil, or beeswax.
- Choose **mineral-based makeup and sunscreens** (zinc oxide or titanium

dioxide) over chemical filters.

Watch out for:

- **Parabens**: mimic estrogen and are linked to hormone disruption.
- **Phthalates**: found in fragrances and plastics, tied to reproductive issues.
- **Formaldehyde & formaldehyde releasers**: carcinogens used in some nail, hair, and body care products.
- **Triclosan**: an antibacterial linked to thyroid disruption and antibiotic resistance.

Switch to Safer Cleaning Products

Why: Common household cleaners often contain harsh chemicals like ammonia, chlorine bleach, and synthetic fragrances that irritate the skin, lungs, and eyes.

What to Do:

- Ditch chemical-heavy products in favor of plant-based brands (look for third-party certifications like *Made Safe*, *EWG Verified*, or *GECA*).
- Make your own cleaners using vinegar, baking soda, and essential oils like tea tree, eucalyptus, or lemon.
- Use HEPA filters and open windows regularly to improve air quality indoors.

Avoid especially:

- **Ammonia**: respiratory irritant, especially risky in unventilated areas.
- **Chlorine bleach**: can react with other cleaners to form toxic gases.
- **Air fresheners and scented candles**: often contain phthalates and undisclosed "fragrance" chemicals that disrupt hormones and linger in

dust.

Read Labels & Use Cleaner Product Guides

Why: Marketing terms like "natural," "clean," and "gentle" are not regulated.
What to Do:

- Use apps and websites like the Environmental Working Group's Skin Deep, Think Dirty, or Chemical Maze to scan products before you buy.
- Avoid long ingredient lists with unrecognizable chemical names, unless verified as safe by trusted databases.

Start Small - Choose One Area for Cleaner Swaps and Build

To minimize waste start buying natural products when you see them on sale and start using them when your product needs to be replaced. Here is a simple guide to use as a plan:

- **Week 1:** Replace your deodorant with a natural or baking soda-based version.
- **Week 2:** Switch to a body wash or soap bar that uses essential oils for fragrance or buy the fragrance-free option.
- **Week 3:** Use your empty surface spray bottle and make a natural version with vinegar, eucalyptus oil and water.
- **Week 2:** Swap plastic water bottles for stainless steel, look for dishwasher safe for convenience and longevity.
- **Week 4:** Swap plastic containers for glass or stainless steel for food

storage.

20

The Body's Detox Dilemma: Natural Systems vs. Synthetic Toxins

Over the past few decades, more than **350,000 chemicals and chemical mixtures** have been registered for production and use globally – a staggering rise documented in the Journal *Environmental Science & Technology* (Wang et al., 2020).

Many in the medical and scientific communities rightly point out that our bodies are equipped with sophisticated natural detoxification systems. The liver, kidneys, lungs, skin, and digestive tract work around the clock to filter, neutralize, and eliminate waste products and harmful substances. But the reality of modern life is that we are now exposed to an unprecedented volume and variety of synthetic chemicals, pollutants and toxins – often at levels that exceed what these natural defenses can handle.

If our bodies were truly adapted to manage this modern chemical onslaught:

- Why have microplastics been detected in the placentas of unborn babies? (Ragusa et al., 2021)
- Why does research show that umbilical cord blood contains, on average, around 300 synthetic chemicals – including many that are known carcinogens or developmental toxins? (Environmental Working Group)

- Why are microplastics accumulating in vital organs – including the liver and brain – with some adults harboring the equivalent of a credit card's worth of plastic in the brain? (Nature Medicine, 2025)
- Why do biomonitoring studies consistently find endocrine-disrupting chemicals such as phthalates, BPA, and PFAS in human blood, urine, and even breast milk? (CDC National Biomonitoring Program)

Today, we are subjected to more environmental and lifestyle toxins than ever before – from heavy metals in fish, pesticides on produce, and microplastics in water and air, to artificial chemicals in processed foods and endocrine disruptors in personal care products. Our bodies, evolved to process naturally occurring toxins, are now grappling with a barrage of synthetic substances that research has linked to hormonal imbalances, neurodevelopmental disorders, immune dysfunction, and certain cancers.

In this chapter, we'll examine the major contributors to modern toxic burden and explore practical, science-based strategies to help reduce exposure and support your body's natural detoxification processes – without fads, extremes, or pseudoscience.

Root Causes of Toxic Load and Detox Dysfunction

In today's world, toxin exposure is nearly unavoidable. From the air we breathe to the food we eat and even the water we drink, chemicals and pathogens quietly accumulate in our bodies. While our liver, gut, kidneys, and lymphatic system are designed to eliminate these toxins, the sheer volume of modern exposures—combined with stress, poor gut health, nutritional deficiencies, and genetics—can overwhelm even the most robust detox system.

Functional practitioners recognize that when detox slows down or becomes dysregulated, it can trigger a cascade of symptoms—fatigue, brain fog, hormonal imbalances, digestive issues, and chronic inflammation. Understanding the hidden contributors to toxic load is the first step in reclaiming your energy, clearing your mind, and supporting true, sustainable healing.

1. Environmental Pollutants

Research suggests we're regularly exposed to hundreds — even thousands — of synthetic chemicals each day, many of which are linked to hormonal imbalances, immune dysfunction, and chronic disease. These toxins enter our bodies through everyday sources:

- **Air Pollution:** Inhaling particulate matter, heavy metals, and volatile organic compounds (VOCs) from traffic, industry, and household products can cause toxin buildup in the lungs and bloodstream.
- **Water Contamination:** Tap water may contain lead, arsenic, pesticides, and industrial chemicals, even after treatment. These accumulate silently over time.
- **Food Sources:** Pesticides, preservatives, artificial colors, and food additives contribute to the daily toxic burden.
- **Household Products:** Everyday items like cleaning agents, plastics, cosmetics, and personal care products can release harmful chemicals such as phthalates, BPA, and parabens, many of which act as endocrine disruptors.

If you've ever experienced skin issues, fatigue, or hormonal imbalances with no clear cause - these invisible exposures may be contributing. For more on how to reduce your exposure, refer to Chapter 19: Reducing Harmful Chemicals - Safer Personal Care, Cleaning, and Food, which discusses safer personal care, cleaning, and dietary choices.

2. Parasites

Parasites are more common than many people realize - especially in those with poor gut health, low stomach acid, or compromised immunity. Exposure can occur through under cooked meat, raw seafood, contaminated fruits and vegetables, or even shared surfaces like doorknobs or bathrooms.

Common symptoms include disrupted sleep, itchy skin, teeth grinding, bloating, digestive issues, and unexplained fatigue.

Parasites contribute to toxicity in several ways:

- **Toxin Release:** Parasites produce metabolic waste that taxes your detox systems.
- **Gut Inflammation:** They damage the intestinal lining, increasing permeability ("leaky gut") and allowing toxins to enter the bloodstream.
- **Immune Strain:** The body's effort to fight them may weaken other areas of detoxification and immune function.

3. Poor Gut Health (Gut Dysbiosis)

A balanced gut microbiome plays a crucial role in detoxification. When disrupted by antibiotics, sugar, stress, or poor diet, harmful bacteria and yeast can overgrow, producing toxic compounds like lipopolysaccharides (LPS) that promote systemic inflammation.

Key concerns related to dysbiosis include:

- **Leaky Gut Syndrome:** When the gut lining becomes inflamed and permeable, toxins, microbes, and undigested food particles can enter the bloodstream, overwhelming the immune system.
- **Impaired Detoxification:** A healthy gut supports liver function, bile flow, and nutrient absorption. Without these, detox slows down significantly.
- **Toxin Re-absorption:** If fiber intake is low or bowel movements are infrequent, toxins eliminated in bile can be reabsorbed—adding to the burden.

If you've experienced food sensitivities, brain fog, or skin flare-ups after eating, it may be your gut trying to send a signal.

4. Poor Liver Function

The liver is your body's main detoxification powerhouse—filtering blood, breaking down toxins, and metabolising hormones. But modern life can overwhelm it. A poor diet, alcohol, medications, and chronic stress all impair liver function.

Signs of a sluggish liver include fatigue, bloating, itchy skin, brain fog, PMS, and difficulty digesting fats.

When the liver slows down:

- **Detoxification stalls:** Toxins and metabolic waste build up, leading to oxidative stress and inflammation.
- **Bile stagnates:** This reduces fat digestion and toxin elimination via the bowel.
- **Hormones recirculate:** Especially estrogen, which can lead to PMS, acne, and estrogen dominance symptoms.

Nourishing your liver through diet, herbs, rest, and reducing toxic exposures can restore its ability to support whole-body health.

5. Mold and Mycotoxins

Often overlooked, exposure to mold and its toxic byproducts (mycotoxins) can cause profound effects on your health. This is especially relevant for anyone who has lived in a water-damaged home, has chronic sinus or respiratory issues, or feels chronically fatigued without explanation.

- **Sources:** Mold can grow behind walls, in air conditioners, bathrooms, or anywhere moisture lingers. Mycotoxins can also be found in contaminated grains, coffee, dried fruits, and nuts.

- **Symptoms:** Brain fog, memory issues, fatigue, allergies, chronic congestion, and mood disturbances.
- **Health Impact:** Mycotoxins suppress the immune system, impair liver function, and disrupt cellular energy production.

Reducing mold exposure, improving indoor air quality, and supporting detox pathways with binders (like activated charcoal or bentonite clay), antioxidants, and glutathione can help recovery.

6. Genetic Variability and Detox Capacity

Not everyone detoxifies at the same rate. Genetic variations such as MTHFR and COMT can slow down the body's ability to eliminate certain toxins—making even low exposures problematic for some individuals.

This means two people with the same lifestyle can have completely different reactions to toxins. If you've always felt extra sensitive to chemicals, fragrances, or medications, these genetic differences might explain why your body needs more support.

Methods of Detoxification

Detoxification is a natural process that the body continuously carries out to remove harmful substances and maintain balance. While detox practices have been used for centuries in traditional medicine, modern research supports their role in promoting health, longevity, and vitality. By integrating effective detox strategies into daily life, individuals can support their liver, digestive system, kidneys, and skin—the primary organs responsible for toxin elimination.

True detoxification doesn't come from a juice cleanse—it starts with a healthy gut and a well-supported liver. These two systems are intimately connected. When your digestion is sluggish or your gut barrier is compromised, your liver becomes overloaded with toxins, waste, and microbial byproducts—including those released by parasites.

In functional medicine, a whole-body cleanse goes beyond short-term detoxes—it involves restoring the gut lining, eliminating hidden infections like parasites, and enhancing your liver's natural detox pathways. For many people, especially those with chronic bloating, fatigue, brain fog, or food sensitivities, addressing gut infections and detox pathways together is the missing piece of the puzzle.

Important Note:

Detoxification should always be approached with care and ideally under the guidance of a qualified health practitioner—especially when addressing parasites, heavy metals, or chronic gut imbalances. The information provided in this chapter is for educational purposes only and is not intended as medical advice or a substitute for personalized care. Every body is different, and attempting to implement all strategies at once may overwhelm your system or trigger unwanted reactions. A skilled practitioner can help you pick and choose a few strategies in accordance to your test results and symptoms, sequencing your protocol steps safely, monitor your progress, and tailor recommendations to your unique needs. Healing is a process—go slow, stay nourished, and listen to your body.

Here are some effective strategies that support detoxification:

Digestive Health & Detoxification

If your gut isn't functioning well, your body simply cannot detox. And if you can't detox, your energy, skin, hormones, and mental clarity will suffer.

Your digestive system isn't just where food is broken down—it's the gatekeeper of your health. It absorbs nutrients, eliminates waste, and plays a critical role in filtering and neutralizing the constant flow of toxins that enter your body through food, air, water, and stress. When this system becomes sluggish, overloaded, or imbalanced, toxins accumulate—leading to inflammation, fatigue, skin issues, brain fog, hormonal imbalances, and chronic disease.

Supporting your digestive health with natural detox aids promotes a thriving microbiome, efficient elimination, and stronger resilience to the toxic load of modern life. Below are evidence-informed, practical strategies to nourish your digestive system and enhance your body's natural detox pathways.

Note: Always work with a qualified health practitioner when undertaking any intensive detoxification program—especially if you are managing chronic illness, taking medications, or are pregnant or breastfeeding. This section is not intended as a one-size-fits-all protocol, but as overarching education to guide informed choices.

Foundational Gut-Supporting Habits

A well-functioning gut is your first line of defense. These simple, daily habits support your body's natural detoxification:

- **Increase Fiber Intake**: Soluble and insoluble fibers found in vegetables, fruits, chia seeds, flaxseeds, and legumes help bind to toxins in the gut and escort them out through healthy bowel movements.
- **Consume Fermented Foods**: Probiotic-rich foods like sauerkraut, kefir, kimchi, and coconut yogurt feed beneficial bacteria, support immune regulation, and crowd out harmful microbes.
- **Hydrate Generously**: Clean, filtered water is essential to keep waste moving and flush out toxins. Aim for at least 1.5 to 2 liters per day, more in warmer climates or during detox protocols.
- **Avoid Processed Foods**: Highly processed and additive-laden foods promote gut dysbiosis and inflammation. Reducing artificial sweeteners, preservatives, seed oils, and synthetic additives lightens the toxic load.
- **Chew Thoroughly**: Digestion begins in the mouth. Chewing food slowly and thoroughly activates digestive enzymes in saliva, easing the burden on the stomach and improving nutrient absorption.

- **Include Natural Digestive Enzymes:** Pineapple, papaya, kiwi, and fermented foods contain enzymes that help break down proteins, fats, and carbohydrates more efficiently.

Intermittent Fasting for a Digestive Reset

Intermittent fasting (IF)—such as the popular 16:8 method, where you fast for 16 hours and eat within an 8-hour window—gives your digestive system a much-needed rest. This pause allows the body to divert energy from constant digestion to deep repair and regeneration. One of the key benefits of fasting is autophagy, a natural "cellular housekeeping" process that helps the body break down damaged cells, misfolded proteins, and intracellular toxins. This can support detoxification, reduce inflammation, and improve mitochondrial function.

From a functional health perspective, IF may help regulate insulin levels, reduce bloating, sharpen mental clarity, and support more balanced gut motility. It can also stimulate the migrating motor complex (MMC)—the wave-like contractions that help sweep debris and bacteria from the small intestine, which is often sluggish in people with digestive issues.

However, intermittent fasting is not for everyone. Women in particular may need a more gentle approach, especially if they're pregnant, breast-feeding, in early postpartum, struggling with adrenal fatigue, underweight, or recovering from disordered eating. In these cases, fasting can further stress the body rather than heal it. Listening to your body's cues, starting slowly, and working with a practitioner are key to ensuring fasting is safe and supportive.

Most importantly, when you are eating, every bite counts. Nutrient density is essential. A fasting routine combined with a poor-quality diet can do more harm than good. Focus on whole, unprocessed foods rich in fiber, antioxidants, healthy fats, protein, and minerals to nourish your cells, support detox pathways, and avoid depletion.

Parasites: The Hidden Saboteurs

Parasites are far more common than we're led to believe—especially in people with low stomach acid, poor gut function, nutrient depletion, or frequent travel. Even without obvious gastrointestinal symptoms, chronic, low-grade parasitic infections can disrupt your microbiome, inflame your gut lining, and drain your energy.

Parasites release neurotoxins and metabolic waste, steal key nutrients (like iron, B12, and zinc), and can contribute to symptoms such as:

- Persistent bloating or gas
- Fatigue that doesn't improve with rest
- Nutrient deficiencies despite a healthy diet
- Teeth grinding, especially at night
- Rashes, itchy skin, or hives
- Sleep disturbances or insomnia
- Intense sugar cravings
- Anal itching (especially in kids)

Mainstream medicine often dismisses the idea of parasites unless symptoms are severe. But in functional and naturopathic circles, addressing parasites is often the first step in resolving stubborn, unexplained symptoms.

Natural Parasite-Cleansing Herbs and Foods

Certain foods and herbs naturally weaken, expel, or inhibit parasites—while supporting gut immunity and microbial balance:

- **Garlic & Onions:** Contain allicin and sulfur compounds with antiparasitic, antifungal, and immune-boosting effects.
- **Pumpkin Seeds:** Contain cucurbitacin, which paralyzes worms and promotes elimination.
- **Papaya Seeds:** Rich in enzymes like carpain, which break down parasite eggs.

- **Fermented Foods:** Help repopulate beneficial bacteria that keep parasites and yeast in check.
- **Coconut Oil:** High in lauric acid, which is anti-fungal and also disrupts parasite membranes.
- **Wormwood, Clove & Black Walnut Hull:** A classic herbal trio used to kill adult worms, larvae, and eggs.
- **Neem & Oregano Oil:** Traditional antimicrobial herbs that purify the gut and blood.
- **Ginger & Turmeric**: Reduce inflammation and help your liver process toxins from parasite die-off.

Start low and slow. As parasites die, they release endotoxins that can trigger a Herxheimer reaction—a short-term flare-up of symptoms like fatigue, brain fog, or headaches. Always support detox pathways (liver, kidneys, bowels, lymph) with proper hydration, rest, and nutrition during any parasite cleanse.

Supporting the Liver

The liver is the body's primary detox organ, processing toxins and waste products to be excreted via the kidneys or intestines. Ensuring liver function remains optimal is crucial for overall well-being contributing to hormonal balance, digestion, metabolizing nutrients and processing toxins. Besides staying hydrated and reducing exposure to alcohol, processed foods, and environmental toxins, prioritizing liver-supportive foods and herbs can make a significant difference, some of these include:

Foods that Support Liver Health

- **Cruciferous Vegetables**: Broccoli, cauliflower, kale, and Brussels sprouts are rich in glucosinolates, which stimulate detoxification enzymes.
- **Garlic and Onions**: High in sulfur compounds, these foods support liver detoxification by enhancing glutathione production.

- **Beets and Carrots**: Their antioxidants and beta-carotene aid in liver repair and reduce oxidative stress.
- **Leafy Greens**: Spinach and arugula neutralize heavy metals and pesticides, reducing liver burden.
- **Healthy Fats**: Avocado, walnuts, and olive oil support cell membrane integrity and liver function.
- **Dandelion tea**: Dandelion tea supports liver health by promoting detoxification, stimulating bile production, and providing antioxidants that protect liver cells from damage.
- **Green Tea**: is a powerful detoxifying beverage, rich in antioxidants, polyphenols, and catechins that enhance the body's natural detox pathways. It primarily supports detoxification by promoting liver function, reducing oxidative stress, and aiding toxin elimination.
- **Flaxseeds and Chia Seeds:** These seeds are high in both soluble and insoluble fiber, making them effective at regulating bowel movements and removing toxins. When soaked in water, they form a gel-like consistency that soothes the digestive tract and helps sweep out the accumulation of waste in the digestive tract.

Advanced Gut-Liver Detox Allies

Supporting detoxification of the liver requires more than "cleansing" foods. The following natural compounds and herbs work synergistically to protect the gut lining, promote toxin elimination, and stimulate liver function: Herbs have long been used to enhance liver function:

- **Milk Thistle**: Milk thistle (*Silybum marianum*) is one of the most well-researched herbs for liver detoxification and overall toxin elimination. Its active compound, silymarin, is a powerful antioxidant that protects and regenerates liver cells, making it essential for supporting the body's natural detox pathways.
- **Dandelion Root**: Dandelion root helps stimulate bile production, which is essential for breaking down fats and eliminating toxins. Bile acts as a

carrier for toxins, ensuring they are excreted through the intestines rather than reabsorbed. Dandelion root increases urine production, which helps flush out toxins, excess salts, and metabolic waste through the kidneys. Unlike synthetic diuretics, it also replenishes potassium, preventing electrolyte imbalances.
- **Schisandra Berry:** Used in Traditional Chinese Medicine for centuries, Schisandra enhances liver function, toxin elimination, and stress resilience, making it a valuable herb for detoxification.
- **Bile-Stimulating Detoxifiers:** Bitter Greens (e.g., dandelion, rocket, endive): Trigger bile flow, which helps carry waste and toxins out of the body.
- **Turmeric (Curcumin):** Enhances bile production and supports phase II liver detox enzymes.
- **Oregano:** Broad-spectrum antimicrobial useful in gut-clearing protocols.

Chlorella & Spirulina: Rich in chlorophyll and antioxidants, these algae help bind heavy metals and support liver detox. Be sure to use clean, third-party tested sources.

Sweating and Saunas

Sweating is one of the body's natural detoxification methods, and saunas have been used for centuries to enhance this process. Regular sauna use, particularly infrared saunas, can help eliminate heavy metals like lead, cadmium, and mercury, as well as environmental toxins such as BPA and phthalates. The heat exposure increases circulation, promoting lymphatic drainage and supporting the liver's detoxification pathways. Studies show that infrared sauna sessions can significantly reduce toxin levels in the body, with one study finding that persistent organic pollutants (POPs) were excreted more effectively through sweat than through urine or faeces.

Additionally, sauna therapy has been linked to improved mitochondrial function, which is essential for energy production and cellular repair.

Beyond detoxification, sauna use has been associated with numerous health benefits, including cardiovascular support, enhanced immune function, reduced arthritis symptoms, better mental well-being, and increased longevity. A 20-year Finnish study found that regular sauna users had a 63% lower risk of sudden cardiac death, and a 40% lower risk of all-cause mortality compared to non-users. Heat exposure triggers a rise in heart rate similar to moderate exercise, improving circulation and vascular health. It also activates heat shock proteins, which reduce inflammation and protect against neurodegenerative diseases such as Alzheimer's. Moreover, sauna use has been shown to improve mood by increasing the release of endorphins and reducing stress hormones like cortisol. Whether used for detoxification or overall well-being, sauna therapy offers a powerful, evidence-backed tool for optimizing health.

For those without access to a sauna, sweating can still be achieved through other methods such as exercise, hot baths, or warm outdoor environments. High-intensity workouts, particularly those that raise the heart rate for extended periods, promote sweating and encourage the body to eliminate toxins through the skin. Studies suggest that moderate aerobic exercise can enhance the body's ability to detoxify through sweat, improving circulation and supporting liver and kidney function. Hot baths with Epsom salts may also stimulate sweating while providing additional detoxification benefits through the absorption of magnesium, which plays a key role in metabolic and detox processes.

Bringing It All Together

Whether you're working on clearing parasites, healing your gut lining, or simply giving your liver some love, the most effective detox protocols:

- Address hidden infections

- Soothe and repair the gut lining
- Stimulate bile flow and toxin elimination
- Use food and herbs as medicine
- Avoid harsh one-size-fits-all "cleanses" that overwhelm the system

You don't need to do everything at once. But by supporting the gut-liver connection, your body becomes more resilient, your energy returns, and long-standing symptoms can begin to shift.

True detoxification isn't about deprivation—it's about nourishment, elimination, and restoration.

21

Benefits of Personalized Nutrition & Health Plans

The real transformations happen with personalized nutrition and health plans tailored to your unique body chemistry, gut microbiome, goals and preferences.

In a world where health advice often feels one-size-fits-all, personalized nutrition emerges as a refreshing, science-backed alternative that caters to your unique needs. Imagine understanding precisely what your body requires to thrive, from optimizing energy levels to preventing chronic diseases. By integrating cutting-edge insights from genetics, lifestyle analysis, and gut health science, personalized nutrition transforms vague dietary guidelines into actionable, tailored strategies. This approach not only enhances physical health but also empowers individuals to take control of their well-being, making each bite a step toward a healthier, more vibrant life. The benefits of personalized nutrition and health plans are as follows:

1. Targeted Nutritional Support

Personalized nutrition allows interventions to be tailored to an individual's unique physiological, genetic, and lifestyle factors, optimizing health outcomes. For example, genetic testing can identify specific nutrient needs, such as increased requirements for omega-3 fatty acids or B vitamins, based on genetic polymorphisms.

2. Improved Dietary Adherence

When nutrition plans are personalized, individuals are more likely to adhere to them. A study found that tailored dietary advice based on genetic and phenotypic data led to better compliance compared to generic recommendations.

3. Enhanced Disease Prevention and Management

Personalized nutrition can help prevent and manage chronic diseases. For instance, individuals with a predisposition to Type 2 diabetes can benefit from targeted dietary interventions, such as reducing carbohydrate intake or focusing on foods with a low glycemic index.

4. Gut Microbiome Optimization

Analyzing the gut microbiome provides insights into dietary adjustments to improve digestion and overall health. Personalized interventions can increase beneficial bacteria, reduce inflammation, and alleviate gastrointestinal symptoms.

5. Better Weight Management

Tailored approaches consider factors like metabolic rate, genetic predisposition, and lifestyle habits, making weight management strategies more effective and sustainable.

6. Improved Mental Health

Personalized diets that target nutritional deficiencies linked to mental health conditions can improve mood and cognitive function. For example, omega-3 fatty acids and folate supplementation have been shown to benefit individuals with depression.

7. Empowerment and Self-Efficacy

By involving individuals in the creation of a nutrition plan based on their data, personalized nutrition fosters a sense of empowerment and ownership over health decisions, leading to more sustainable behavior changes.

8. Reduction in Unnecessary Supplements

Personalized nutrition helps identify specific deficiencies, reducing the need for broad-spectrum supplements and focusing only on necessary nutrients. This approach is both cost-effective and reduces the risk of over-supplementation.

Test Don't Guess – Functional Tests

Gut microbiome and Hair Tissue Mineral Analysis (HTMA) tests are two of the most valuable functional health assessments because they provide in-depth, personalized insights into key areas of your health that often go unnoticed but are critical to restoring your energy and vitality.

While a gut microbiome test focuses on digestion, immunity, and nutrient absorption, HTMA examines your body's mineral balance and toxic load. Together, they provide a comprehensive picture of your internal health. Addressing both gut health and mineral imbalances ensures that your body can effectively process nutrients and maintain a healthy metabolism, improving your energy and overall well-being.

Many chronic health issues, such as persistent fatigue or bloating, can be traced back to gut imbalances. By identifying the specific bacteria that are either missing or overgrown, you can make targeted dietary and lifestyle changes, helping to restore balance, boost energy, and improve overall well-being.

Both tests provide highly personalized insights. They don't just offer a diagnosis; they provide clear, actionable steps to help you restore balance. This is especially important for busy mothers who need practical solutions to regain their energy and vitality.

Look for a qualified expert with extensive experience with interpreting these tests and a track record of achieving results for their clients.

Gut Microbiome Testing

The gut microbiome is central to so many aspects of health, from digestion and nutrient absorption to immune function and mood regulation. Poor gut health can lead to a range of symptoms, including fatigue, brain fog, digestive issues, and weakened immunity. By assessing the diversity and balance of bacteria in your gut, this test helps you understand how well your body is processing nutrients and fighting off illness, which directly affects your energy levels.

Many gut microbiome tests can help address the following:

1. **Digestive Health and Nutrient Absorption**

A gut microbiome test can show if you have the right balance of bacteria to help digest food and absorb nutrients efficiently. If you're lacking certain beneficial bacteria, your body might not be absorbing vital vitamins and minerals like iron, B vitamins, and magnesium properly—nutrients that are essential for energy and reducing fatigue.

1. **Immune System Support**

Feeling constantly run down can be a sign that your immune system is struggling. Since most of your immune function is based in your gut, an imbalance in your microbiome could make you more prone to illness or chronic low-grade inflammation, which can sap your energy.

1. **Hormonal and Mood Balance**

Your gut produces important neurotransmitters, like serotonin, that regulate mood and energy levels. A microbiome test may reveal whether your gut is supporting or hindering this process. If your gut is inflamed or imbalanced, it can affect not only your digestion but also your mood and mental clarity, contributing to feelings of fatigue or overwhelm.

1. **Chronic Fatigue and Energy Regulation**

Poor gut health can lead to insulin resistance, blood sugar imbalances, and even chronic inflammation, all of which drain your energy and leave you feeling tired no matter how much sleep you get. Identifying these imbalances through a test can help you understand why you might be experiencing brain fog, energy crashes, or overall sluggishness.

1. **Food Intolerances and Sensitivities**

If you're feeling bloated, sluggish, or uncomfortable after meals, it might be due to food sensitivities that can disrupt your gut health. A microbiome test can highlight potential issues with gluten, dairy, or other foods that might be contributing to inflammation or digestive issues, causing you to feel tired and depleted.

1. **Personalized Diet Recommendations**

With test results in hand, you can tailor your diet to include foods that nourish the beneficial bacteria in your gut, helping restore balance and improve energy. Simple changes like incorporating more fiber, prebiotic-rich foods, and reducing processed foods can make a big difference in how you feel day-to-day.

Hair Tissue Mineral Analysis (HTMA) Tests

Hair Tissue Mineral Analysis (HTMA) is another valuable tool for understanding the underlying reasons why you might be feeling exhausted, run down, or out of balance. This non-invasive test analyses the mineral content of your hair, providing a detailed look at your body's long-term mineral status and revealing potential heavy metal toxicity. For mothers who are constantly tired, HTMA can offer insights into your body's mineral stores and help identify deficiencies or imbalances that could be affecting your energy and health. HTMA tests can help address the following:

1. **Mineral Deficiencies and Fatigue**

Minerals like magnesium, iron, calcium, and zinc play critical roles in energy production, muscle and hormone function, and overall vitality. If you're constantly feeling tired, an HTMA test can reveal whether your mineral levels are too low, which could be draining your energy. For instance, magnesium is crucial for reducing stress and supporting sleep, while iron is vital for transporting oxygen throughout your body.

1. **Heavy Metal Toxicity and Health Impact**

Exposure to heavy metals such as mercury, lead, aluminum, or cadmium can disrupt your body's natural processes which can severely impact your health, leading to fatigue, brain fog, and weakened immunity. These metals can accumulate in the body over time, leading to fatigue, brain fog, and hormonal imbalances. Identifying and reducing your exposure to these toxins is crucial for regaining energy and supporting long-term health. HTMA tests can detect the presence of these toxic metals, allowing you to take steps to reduce exposure and support your body in detoxifying them.

1. **Chronic Stress and Hormonal Imbalances**

Stress depletes your body of essential minerals, like magnesium and calcium, making it harder to cope with the daily pressures of life. HTMA can reveal the impact of chronic stress on your mineral levels, which in turn can influence how well you handle physical and emotional demands. Balancing these minerals through diet and supplementation can help you feel more resilient and improve your mood and energy levels.

1. **Metabolic and Thyroid Function**

Your mineral levels are closely tied to your thyroid and adrenal health, which regulate your metabolism and energy. An HTMA test can highlight imbalances in minerals such as iodine and selenium, which are key for thyroid function. Addressing these imbalances can improve your metabolism, reduce fatigue, and help you maintain a healthy weight.

1. **Bone Health and Muscle Function**

HTMA can show whether minerals like boron, calcium and magnesium are in balance to support your bone density and muscle strength. If you're deficient, you may be more prone to aches, pains, and fatigue, and knowing this allows you to make targeted improvements through your diet and lifestyle.

1. **Customized Nutritional Support**

One of the most beneficial aspects of HTMA is the ability to receive personalized recommendations based on your unique mineral profile. With these insights, you can make changes to your diet or add specific supplements to restore balance, improve energy, and support long-term health. This can be particularly helpful for mothers, as we often experience nutrient depletion due to stress, pregnancy, and breastfeeding.

By addressing both mineral deficiencies and potential heavy metal toxicity, HTMA tests provide a clearer picture of your overall health and help you make informed decisions to restore balance. For a busy mom, understanding and correcting these imbalances can be key to feeling more energized, focused, and ready to take on the demands of daily life.

22

Conclusion

Moving Forward with Confidence: Thriving in Motherhood

Motherhood is a profound transformation – physically, mentally, and emotionally. Yet, in a world that often glorifies bouncing back rather than replenishing, too many mothers are left depleted, struggling with fatigue, brain fog, hormonal imbalances, and a sense of overwhelm. This book has shown that postnatal depletion is not just a phase to endure, but a condition that can be recognized, addressed, and healed through nutrition, lifestyle shifts, and self-care practices. By understanding the intricate connections between gut health, hormone balance, nutrient repletion, and mental well-being, mothers can reclaim their vitality, strength, and joy.

As you can see after reading this book, everything is interrelated, and this is why a holistic approach to healing and vitality is essential. It involves nurturing the mind, body, and spirit through a combination of mindfulness, stress management, balanced nutrition, reducing your toxic load, adequate rest, and avoiding harmful chemicals. By embracing these strategies, new mothers can enhance their recovery, boost their energy levels, and achieve a greater sense of well-being during this transformative period.

Healing from postnatal depletion and optimizing your health is not about perfection – it's about consistent, nourishing choices that support both body and mind. Prioritizing whole, nutrient-dense foods, restorative sleep, mindful movement, and gut-supporting habits will allow you to rebuild your energy reserves and thrive. Your health is not only essential for you but also for your children, your relationships, and your overall quality of life.

Motherhood is not meant to be lived in survival mode. With the right tools, knowledge, and self-compassion, you can emerge from depletion stronger, more resilient, and deeply nourished. The journey back to vitality may take time, but each small step – each nourishing meal, each deep breath, each moment of rest – is a step toward lasting well-being. You are not alone in this, and you are more capable than you know.

Here's to thriving – not just surviving – through motherhood.

Scientific References

The information presented in this book is based on a selection of scientific studies and reputable sources, which have been carefully reviewed and incorporated into the content. While this is not an exhaustive list of all the research used in the development of this book, it serves as a foundation for the evidence-based insights shared. Readers are encouraged to explore these references further as part of their own independent research journey to deepen their understanding of the topics discussed.

Introduction

1. Aparicio, E., Jardí, C., Bedmar, C., Pallejà, M., Basora, J., Arija, V., & The Eclipses Study Group (2020). Nutrient Intake during Pregnancy and Post-Partum: ECLIPSES Study. Nutrients, 12(5), 1325. https://doi.org/10.3390/nu12051325
2. Cleveland Clinic. (2022). Postpartum depression: Types, symptoms, treatment & prevention. Cleveland Clinic. https://my.clevelandclinic.org/health/diseases/9312-postpartum-depression
3. Godfrey, K. M., et al. (2023). Maternal B-vitamin and vitamin D status before, during, and after pregnancy and the influence of supplementation preconception and during pregnancy: Prespecified secondary analysis of the NiPPeR double-blind randomized controlled trial. PLOS Medicine. doi.org/10.1371/journal.pmed.1004260.
4. Shorey, S., Chee, C. Y. I., Ng, E. D., Chan, Y. H., Tam, W. W. S., & Chong, Y. S. (2018). Prevalence and incidence of postpartum depression among healthy mothers: A systematic review and meta-analysis. Journal of psychiatric research, 104, 235–248. https://doi.org/10.1016/j.jpsych

ires.2018.08.001Tosto, V., Ceccobelli, M., Lucarini, E., Tortorella, A., Gerli, S., Parazzini, F., & Favilli, A. (2023). Maternity Blues: A Narrative Review. Journal of personalized medicine, 13(1), 154. https://doi.org/10.3390/jpm13010154

5. Carlson K, Mughal S, Azhar Y, et al. Perinatal Depression. [Updated 2025 Jan 22]. In: StatPearls [Internet]. Treasure Island (FL): StatPearls Publishing; 2025 Jan-. Available from: https://www.ncbi.nlm.nih.gov/books/NBK519070/

6. Rezaie-Keikhaie, K., Arbabshastan, M. E., Rafiemanesh, H., Amirshahi, M., Ostadkelayeh, S. M., & Arbabisarjou, A. (2020). Systematic Review and Meta-Analysis of the Prevalence of the Maternity Blues in the Postpartum Period. Journal of Obstetric, Gynecologic & Neonatal Nursing, 49(2), 127–136. https://doi.org/10.1016/j.jogn.2020.01.001

7. Kiani, A. K., Dhuli, K., Donato, K., Aquilanti, B., Velluti, V., Matera, G., Iaconelli, A., Connelly, S. T., Bellinato, F., Gisondi, P., & Bertelli, M. (2022). Main nutritional deficiencies. Journal of preventive medicine and hygiene, 63(2 Suppl 3), E93–E101. https://doi.org/10.15167/2421-4248/jpmh2022.63.2S3.2752

8. Zielińska, M., Łuszczki, E., & Dereń, K. (2023). Dietary Nutrient Deficiencies and Risk of Depression (Review Article 2018-2023). Nutrients, 15(11), 2433. https://doi.org/10.3390/nu15112433

9. Georgieff, M. K., Ramel, S. E., & Cusick, S. E. (2018). Nutritional influences on brain development. Acta paediatrica (Oslo, Norway: 1992), 107(8), 1310–1321. https://doi.org/10.1111/apa.14287

10. Wachs, T. D. (2009). Models linking nutritional deficiencies to maternal and child mental health. The American Journal of Clinical Nutrition, 89(3), 935S939S. https://doi.org/10.3945/ajcn.2008.26692b

11. Nattagh-Eshtivani, E., Sani, M. A., Dahri, M., Ghalichi, F., Ghavami, A., Arjang, P., & Tarighat-Esfanjani, A. (2018). The role of nutrients in the pathogenesis and treatment of migraine headaches: Review. Biomedicine & Pharmacotherapy, 102, 317–325. https://doi.org/10.1016/j.biopha.2018.03.059

12. Mendiratta, V., Rana, S., Jassi, R., & Chander, R. (2019). Study of

Causative Factors and Clinical Patterns of Periorbital Pigmentation. Indian dermatology online journal, 10(3), 293–295. https://doi.org/10.4103/idoj.IDOJ_158_18

13. Barnish, M., Sheikh, M., & Scholey, A. (2023). Nutrient Therapy for the Improvement of Fatigue Symptoms. Nutrients, 15(9), 2154. https://doi.org/10.3390/nu15092154

14. Álvarez-Herms, J., González, A., Corbi, F., Odriozola, I., & Odriozola, A. (2023). Possible relationship between the gut leaky syndrome and musculoskeletal injuries: the important role of gut microbiota as indirect modulator. AIMS public health, 10(3), 710–738. https://doi.org/10.3934/publichealth.2023049

15. National Institute of Health. (2017). Office of Dietary Supplements - Biotin. Nih.gov. https://ods.od.nih.gov/factsheets/Biotin-HealthProfessional/

16. Chhabra, S., Chhabra, N., Kaur, A., & Gupta, N. (2017). Wound Healing Concepts in Clinical Practice of OMFS. Journal of maxillofacial and oral surgery, 16(4), 403–423. https://doi.org/10.1007/s12663-016-0880-z

17. Guo, S., & Dipietro, L. A. (2010). Factors affecting wound healing. Journal of dental research, 89(3), 219–229. https://doi.org/10.1177/0022034509359125

18. Australian Institute of Health and Welfare. (2012, July 3). Perinatal depression: data from the 2010 Australian National Infant Feeding Survey, Summary. Australian Institute of Health and Welfare. https://www.aihw.gov.au/reports/primary-health-care/perinatal-depression-data-from-the-2010-australia/summary

19. Tal R, Taylor HS. Endocrinology of Pregnancy. [Updated 2021 Mar 18]. In: Feingold KR, Anawalt B, Blackman MR, et al., editors. Endotext [Internet]. South Dartmouth (MA): MDText.com, Inc.; 2000-. Available from: https://www.ncbi.nlm.nih.gov/books/NBK278962/

What is Postnatal Depletion?

1. Campbell, S. A., Dys, S. P., Henderson, T., Bradley, H. A., & Rucklidge,

J. J. (2024). Exploring the impact of antenatal micronutrients used as a treatment for maternal depression on infant temperament in the first year of life. Frontiers in Nutrition, 11. https://doi.org/10.3389/fnut.2024.1307701

2. Carlson K, Mughal S, Azhar Y, et al. Perinatal Depression. [Updated 2025 Jan 22]. In: StatPearls [Internet]. Treasure Island (FL): StatPearls Publishing; 2025 Jan-. Available from: https://www.ncbi.nlm.nih.gov/books/NBK519070/

3. Deligiannidis, K. M., & Freeman, M. P. (2014). Complementary and alternative medicine therapies for perinatal depression. Best practice & research. Clinical obstetrics & gynaecology, 28(1), 85–95. https://doi.org/10.1016/j.bpobgyn.2013.08.007

4. Dye, C., Lenz, K. M., & Leuner, B. (2022). Immune System Alterations and Postpartum Mental Illness: Evidence from Basic and Clinical Research. Frontiers in global women's health, 2, 758748. https://doi.org/10.3389/fgwh.2021.758748

5. Fall, C. H., Sachdev, H. S., Osmond, C., Restrepo-Mendez, M. C., Victora, C., Martorell, R., Stein, A. D., Sinha, S., Tandon, N., Adair, L., Bas, I., Norris, S., Richter, L. M., & COHORTS investigators (2015). Association between maternal age at childbirth and child and adult outcomes in the offspring: a prospective study in five low-income and middle-income countries (COHORTS collaboration). The Lancet. Global health, 3(7), e366–e377. https://doi.org/10.1016/S2214-109X(15)00038-8

6. Fish-Williamson, A., & Hahn-Holbrook, J. (2023). Nutritional factors and cross-national postpartum depression prevalence: an updated meta-analysis and meta-regression of 412 studies from 46 countries. Frontiers in psychiatry, 14, 1193490. https://doi.org/10.3389/fpsyt.2023.1193490

7. Guo, E. L., & Katta, R. (2017). Diet and hair loss: effects of nutrient deficiency and supplement use. Dermatology practical & conceptual, 7(1), 1–10. https://doi.org/10.5826/dpc.0701a01

8. Guo, S., & Dipietro, L. A. (2010). Factors affecting wound healing. Journal of dental research, 89(3), 219–229. https://doi.org/10.1177/002203450

9359125

9. Hall, K., Evans, J., Roberts, R. et al. Mothers' accounts of the impact of being in nature on postnatal well-being: a focus group study. BMC Women's Health 23, 32 (2023). https://doi.org/10.1186/s12905-023-02165-x

10. Hung, M., Blazejewski, A., Lee, S., Lu, J., Soto, A., Schwartz, C. and Amir Mohajeri (2024). Nutritional Deficiencies and Associated Oral Health in Adolescents: A Comprehensive Scoping Review. Children, 11(7), pp.869–869. doi: https://doi.org/10.3390/children11070869

11. King J. C. (2003). The risk of maternal nutritional depletion and poor outcomes increases in early or closely spaced pregnancies. The Journal of nutrition, 133(5 Suppl 2), 1732S–1736S. https://doi.org/10.1093/jn/133.5.1732S

12. Kozlak, S. T., Walsh, S. J., & Lalla, R. V. (2010). Reduced dietary intake of vitamin B12 and folate in patients with recurrent aphthous stomatitis. Journal of oral pathology & medicine: official publication of the International Association of Oral Pathologists and the American Academy of Oral Pathology, 39(5), 420–423. https://doi.org/10.1111/j.1600-0714.2009.00867.x

13. Lu, X., Shi, Z., Jiang, L., & Zhang, S. (2024). Maternal gut microbiota in the health of mothers and offspring: from the perspective of immunology. Frontiers in immunology, 15, 1362784. https://doi.org/10.3389/fimmu.2024.1362784

14. Naidu, R. (2021). Chemical pollution: A growing peril and potential catastrophic risk to humanity. Environment International, 156(106616), 106616. https://doi.org/10.1016/j.envint.2021.106616Knox, B., Galera, C., Sutter-Dallay, A. L., Heude, B., de Lauzon-Guillain, B., & van der Waerden, J. (2023). A network analysis of nutritional markers and maternal perinatal mental health in the French EDEN cohort. BMC pregnancy and childbirth, 23(1), 603. https://doi.org/10.1186/s12884-023-05914-w

15. Pattnaik, H., Mir, M., Boike, S., Kashyap, R., Khan, S. A., & Surani, S. (2022). Nutritional Elements in Sleep. Cureus, 14(12), e32803. https://d

oi.org/10.7759/cureus.32803

16. Rodrigo Barbano Weingrill, Lee, M., Benny, P., Riel, J. M., Saiki, K., Garcia, J., de, L., Fonseca, S., Souza, S. T., Felicetta D'Amato, Uéslen Rocha Silva, Dutra, S., Marques, X., Alexandre Urban Borbely, & Johann Urschitz. (2023). Temporal trends in microplastic accumulation in placentas from pregnancies in Hawai'i. Environment International, 180, 108220–108220. https://doi.org/10.1016/j.envint.2023.108220

17. Ross, K.M., Dunkel Schetter, C., Carroll, J.E., Mancuso, R.A., Breen, E.C., Okun, M.L., Hobel, C. and Coussons-Read, M. (2022). Inflammatory and immune marker trajectories from pregnancy to one-year post-birth. Cytokine, 149, p.155758. doi: https://doi.org/10.1016/j.cyto.2021.155758

18. Tapalaga, G., Bumbu, B. A., Reddy, S. R., Vutukuru, S. D., Nalla, A., Bratosin, F., Fericean, R. M., Dumitru, C., Crisan, D. C., Nicolae, N., & Luca, M. M. (2023). The Impact of Prenatal Vitamin D on Enamel Defects and Tooth Erosion: A Systematic Review. Nutrients, 15(18), 3863. https://doi.org/10.3390/nu15183863

19. Trifu, S., Vladuti, A., & Popescu, A. (2019). THE NEUROENDOCRINOLOGICAL ASPECTS OF PREGNANCY AND POSTPARTUM DEPRESSION. Acta endocrinologica (Bucharest, Romania: 2005), 15(3), 410–415. https://doi.org/10.4183/aeb.2019.410

20. Vora, R. V., Gupta, R., Mehta, M. J., Chaudhari, A. H., Pilani, A. P., & Patel, N. (2014). Pregnancy and skin. Journal of family medicine and primary care, 3(4), 318–324. https://doi.org/10.4103/2249-4863.148099

21. We, J. S., Han, K., Kwon, H. S., & Kil, K. (2018). Effect of Childbirth Age on Bone Mineral Density in Postmenopausal Women. Journal of Korean medical science, 33(48), e311. https://doi.org/10.3346/jkms.2018.33.e311

Nutritional Replenishment to Overcome Deficiencies

1. Accortt, E. E., Lamb, A., Mirocha, J., & Hobel, C. J. (2018). Vitamin D deficiency and depressive symptoms in pregnancy are associated

with adverse perinatal outcomes. Journal of behavioral medicine, 41(5), 680–689. https://doi.org/10.1007/s10865-018-9924-9
2. Batalha, M. A., dos Reis Costa, P. N., Ferreira, A. L. L., Freitas-Costa, N. C., Figueiredo, A. C. C., Shahab-Ferdows, S., Hampel, D., Allen, L. H., Pérez-Escamilla, R., & Kac, G. (2022). Maternal Mental Health in Late Pregnancy and Longitudinal Changes in Postpartum Serum Vitamin B-12, Homocysteine, and Milk B-12 Concentration Among Brazilian Women. Frontiers in Nutrition, 9. https://doi.org/10.3389/fnut.2022.923569
3. Bradley, M., Melchor, J., Carr, R., & Karjoo, S. (2023). Obesity and malnutrition in children and adults: A clinical review. Obesity Pillars, 8, 100087–100087. https://doi.org/10.1016/j.obpill.2023.100087
4. Dowlati, Y., Ravindran, A. V., Segal, Z. V., Stewart, D. E., Steiner, M., & Meyer, J. H. (2017). Selective dietary supplementation in early postpartum is associated with high resilience against depressed mood. Proceedings of the National Academy of Sciences of the United States of America, 114(13), 3509–3514. https://doi.org/10.1073/pnas.1611965114
5. Etebary, S., Nikseresht, S., Sadeghipour, H. R., & Zarrindast, M. R. (2010). Postpartum depression and role of serum trace elements. Iranian journal of psychiatry, 5(2), 40–46.
6. Field, D. T., Cracknell, R. O., Eastwood, J. R., Scarfe, P., Williams, C. M., Zheng, Y., & Tavassoli, T. (2022). High-dose Vitamin B6 supplementation reduces anxiety and strengthens visual surround suppression. Human Psychopharmacology: Clinical and Experimental, 37(6). https://doi.org/10.1002/hup.2852
7. Ghorbani, Ahmad & Darmani kuhi, Hassan & Mohit, Ardeshir. (2013). A review Hair tissue analysis: An analytical method for determining essential elements, toxic elements, hormones and drug use and abuse. International Research Journal of Applied and Basic Sciences. 4. 3675-3688.
8. Godfrey, K. M., Titcombe, P., El-Heis, S., Albert, B. B., Elizabeth Huiwen Tham, Barton, S. J., Kenealy, T., Mary Foong-Fong Chong, Nield, H., Yap Seng Chong, Chan, S.-Y., & Cutfield, W. S. (2023). Maternal B-

vitamin and vitamin D status before, during, and after pregnancy and the influence of supplementation preconception and during pregnancy: Prespecified secondary analysis of the NiPPeR double-blind randomized controlled trial. PLOS Medicine, 20(12), e1004260–e1004260. https://doi.org/10.1371/journal.pmed.1004260

9. Gropper S. S. (2023). The Role of Nutrition in Chronic Disease. Nutrients, 15(3), 664. https://doi.org/10.3390/nu15030664

10. Heidelbaugh J. J. (2013). Proton pump inhibitors and risk of vitamin and mineral deficiency: evidence and clinical implications. Therapeutic advances in drug safety, 4(3), 125–133. https://doi.org/10.1177/2042098613482484

11. Kang, D. W., & DiBaise, J. K. (2012). Effects of gut microbes on nutrient absorption and energy regulation. Nutrition in clinical practice: official publication of the American Society for Parenteral and Enteral Nutrition, 27(2), 201–214. https://doi.org/10.1177/0884533611436116

12. Lin, Y. H., Chen, C. M., Su, H. M., Mu, S. C., Chang, M. L., Chu, P. Y., & Li, S. C. (2019). Association between Postpartum Nutritional Status and Postpartum Depression Symptoms. Nutrients, 11(6), 1204. https://doi.org/10.3390/nu11061204

13. Martini, D., Godos, J., Bonaccio, M., Vitaglione, P., & Grosso, G. (2021). Ultra-Processed Foods and Nutritional Dietary Profile: A Meta-Analysis of Nationally Representative Samples. Nutrients, 13(10), 3390. https://doi.org/10.3390/nu13103390

14. National Institutes of Health (NIH). (2024). Vitamin K. https://ods.od.nih.gov/factsheets/VitaminK-HealthProfessional/

15. Park, S. B., Choi, S. W., & Nam, A. Y. (2009). Hair Tissue Mineral Analysis and Metabolic Syndrome. Biological Trace Element Research, 130(3), 218–228. https://doi.org/10.1007/s12011-009-8336-7

16. Shetty, S. S., D, D., S, H., Sonkusare, S., Naik, P. B., Kumari N, S., & Madhyastha, H. (2023). Environmental pollutants and their effects on human health. Heliyon, 9(9), e19496. https://doi.org/10.1016/j.heliyon.2023.e19496

17. Singh, S., Kumar, V., Gill, J. P. K., Datta, S., Singh, S., Dhaka, V., Kapoor,

D., Wani, A. B., Dhanjal, D. S., Kumar, M., Harikumar, S. L., & Singh, J. (2020). Herbicide Glyphosate: Toxicity and Microbial Degradation. International journal of environmental research and public health, 17(20), 7519. https://doi.org/10.3390/ijerph17207519
18. Susič, D., Bombač Tavčar, L., Lučovnik, M., Hrobat, H., Gornik, L., & Gradišek, A. (2023). Wellbeing Forecasting in Postpartum Anemia Patients. Healthcare (Basel, Switzerland), 11(12), 1694. https://doi.org/10.3390/healthcare11121694
19. Tardy, A. L., Pouteau, E., Marquez, D., Yilmaz, C., & Scholey, A. (2020). Vitamins and Minerals for Energy, Fatigue and Cognition: A Narrative Review of the Biochemical and Clinical Evidence. Nutrients, 12(1), 228. https://doi.org/10.3390/nu12010228
20. Zhang, MM., Zou, Y., Li, SM. et al. The efficacy and safety of omega-3 fatty acids on depressive symptoms in perinatal women: a meta-analysis of randomized placebo-controlled trials. Transl Psychiatry 10, 193 (2020). https://doi.org/10.1038/s41398-020-00886-3

Eating to Fight Chronic Inflammation

1. Ambreen, G., Siddiq, A., & Hussain, K. (2020). Association of long-term consumption of repeatedly heated mix vegetable oils in different doses and hepatic toxicity through fat accumulation. Lipids in health and disease, 19(1), 69. https://doi.org/10.1186/s12944-020-01256-0
2. Brookes G. (2022). Genetically Modified (GM) Crop Use 1996-2020: Environmental Impacts Associated with Pesticide Use CHANGE. GM crops & food, 13(1), 262–289. https://doi.org/10.1080/21645698.2022.2118497
3. Chen, W. Y., Fu, Y. P., Zhong, W., & Zhou, M. (2021). The Association Between Dietary Inflammatory Index and Sex Hormones Among Post-menopausal Women in the US. Frontiers in endocrinology, 12, 771565. https://doi.org/10.3389/fendo.2021.771565
4. Dandona, P., Aljada, A., & Bandyopadhyay, A. (2004). Inflammation: the link between insulin resistance, obesity and diabetes. Trends in

immunology, 25(1), 4–7. https://doi.org/10.1016/j.it.2003.10.013
5. DiNicolantonio, J. J., & O'Keefe, J. H. (2018). Omega-6 vegetable oils as a driver of coronary heart disease: the oxidized linoleic acid hypothesis. Open heart, 5(2), e000898. https://doi.org/10.1136/openhrt-2018-000898
6. Furman, D., Campisi, J., Verdin, E., Carrera-Bastos, P., Targ, S., Franceschi, C., Ferrucci, L., & Slavich, G. M. (2019). Chronic inflammation in the etiology of disease across the life span. Nature Medicine, 25(12), 1822–1832. https://doi.org/10.1038/s41591-019-0675-0
7. GBD 2017 Diet Collaborators (2019). Health effects of dietary risks in 195 countries, 1990-2017: a systematic analysis for the Global Burden of Disease Study 2017. Lancet (London, England), 393(10184), 1958–1972. https://doi.org/10.1016/S0140-6736(19)30041-8
8. Gharby S. (2022). Refining Vegetable Oils: Chemical and Physical Refining. TheScientificWorldJournal, 2022, 6627013. https://doi.org/10.1155/2022/6627013
9. Hu, F. B., & Malik, V. S. (2010). Sugar-sweetened beverages and risk of obesity and type 2 diabetes: epidemiologic evidence. Physiology & behavior, 100(1), 47–54. https://doi.org/10.1016/j.physbeh.2010.01.036
10. Innes, J. K., & Calder, P. C. (2018). Omega-6 fatty acids and inflammation. Prostaglandins, leukotrienes, and essential fatty acids, 132, 41–48. https://doi.org/10.1016/j.plefa.2018.03.004
11. Lerner, A., Benzvi, C. and Aristo Vojdani (2024). Gluten is a Proinflammatory Inducer of Autoimmunity. Journal of Translational Gastroenterology, [online] 2(2), pp.109–124. doi: https://doi.org/10.14218/jtg.2023.00060
12. Macdonald I. A. (2016). A review of recent evidence relating to sugars, insulin resistance and diabetes. European journal of nutrition, 55(Suppl 2), 17–23. https://doi.org/10.1007/s00394-016-1340-8
13. Maral Bishehkolaei, & Pathak, Y. (2024). Influence of Omega n-6/n-3 Ratio on Cardiovascular Disease and Nutritional interventions. Human

Nutrition & Metabolism, 37, 200275–200275. https://doi.org/10.1016/j.hnm.2024.200275

14. Pahwa R, Goyal A, Jialal I. Chronic Inflammation. [Updated 2023 Aug 7]. In: StatPearls [Internet]. Treasure Island (FL): StatPearls Publishing; 2025 Jan-. Available from: https://www.ncbi.nlm.nih.gov/books/NBK493173/

15. Philip, A., & White, N. D. (2022). Gluten, Inflammation, and Neurodegeneration. American journal of lifestyle medicine, 16(1), 32–35. https://doi.org/10.1177/15598276211049345

16. Scheiber A, Mank V. Anti-Inflammatory Diets. [Updated 2023 Oct 28]. In: StatPearls [Internet]. Treasure Island (FL): StatPearls Publishing; 2025 Jan-. Available from: https://www.ncbi.nlm.nih.gov/books/NBK597377/

17. Sears, B., & Saha, A. K. (2021). Dietary Control of Inflammation and Resolution. Frontiers in nutrition, 8, 709435. https://doi.org/10.3389/fnut.2021.709435

18. Statista. (2023, June 13). U.S. canola oil consumption, 2021. Retrieved from Statista website: https://www.statista.com/statistics/301036/canola-oil-consumption-united-states/

19. Szandra Klátyik, Simon, G., Oláh, M., Mesnage, R., Antoniou, M. N., Zaller, J. G., & András Székács. (2023). Terrestrial ecotoxicity of glyphosate, its formulations, and co-formulants: evidence from 2010–2023. Environ Sci Eur, 35(1). https://doi.org/10.1186/s12302-023-00758-9

20. U.S. Food and Drug Administration. (2022). GMO crops, animal food, and beyond. GMO Crops, Animal Food, and Beyond. Retrieved from https://www.fda.gov/food/agricultural-biotechnology/gmo-crops-animal-food-and-beyond

21. Van Zonneveld, S. M., van den Oever, E. J., Haarman, B. C. M., Grandjean, E. L., Nuninga, J. O., van de Rest, O., & Sommer, I. E. C. (2024). An Anti-Inflammatory Diet and Its Potential Benefit for Individuals with Mental Disorders and Neurodegenerative Diseases-A Narrative Review. Nutrients, 16(16), 2646. https://doi.org/10.3390/nu16162646

22. Xia, Q., Du, Z., Lin, D., Huo, L., Qin, L., Wang, W., ... An, Y. (2021). Review on contaminants in edible oil and analytical technologies. Oil Crop Science, 6(1), 23–27. https://doi.org/10.1016/j.ocsci.2021.02.001
23. Yamashima, T., Ota, T., Mizukoshi, E., Nakamura, H., Yamamoto, Y., Kikuchi, M., Yamashita, T., & Kaneko, S. (2020). Intake of ω-6 Polyunsaturated Fatty Acid-Rich Vegetable Oils and Risk of Lifestyle Diseases. Advances in nutrition (Bethesda, Md.), 11(6), 1489–1509
24. Zielinski, M. R., Systrom, D. M., & Rose, N. R. (2019). Fatigue, Sleep, and Autoimmune and Related Disorders. Frontiers in immunology, 10, 1827. https://doi.org/10.3389/fimmu.2019.01827

The Postpartum Hormonal Roller-coaster

1. Alur-Gupta, S., Boland, M. R., Barnhart, K. T., Sammel, M. D., & Dokras, A. (2021). Postpartum complications increased in women with polycystic ovary syndrome. *American journal of obstetrics and gynecology*, 224(3), 280.e1–280.e13. https://doi.org/10.1016/j.ajog.2020.08.048
2. American College of Obstetricians and Gynecologists. (2018). Postpartum depression. Retrieved from https://www.acog.org
3. Anderson, G. H., & Moore, S. E. (2004). "Dietary proteins in the regulation of food intake and body weight in humans." The Journal of Nutrition, 134(4), 974S-979S. https://doi.org/10.1093/jn/134.4.974S
4. Aziz, T., Hussain, N., Hameed, Z., & Lin, L. (2024). Elucidating the role of diet in maintaining gut health to reduce the risk of obesity, cardiovascular and other age-related inflammatory diseases: recent challenges and future recommendations. *Gut microbes*, 16(1), 2297864. https://doi.org/10.1080/19490976.2023.2297864
5. Bafkar, N., Zeraattalab-Motlagh, S., Jayedi, A. *et al.* Efficacy and safety of omega-3 fatty acids supplementation for anxiety symptoms: a systematic review and dose-response meta-analysis of randomized controlled trials. *BMC Psychiatry* **24**, 455 (2024). https://doi.org/10.1186/s12888-024-05881-2
6. Banaei, M., Azizi, M., Moridi, A. *et al.* Sexual dysfunction and related

factors in pregnancy and postpartum: a systematic review and meta-analysis protocol. *Syst Rev* **8**, 161 (2019). https://doi.org/10.1186/s13643-019-1079-4

7. Bikle, D. (2014). "Vitamin D metabolism, mechanism of action, and clinical applications." Chemistry & Biology, 21(3), 319-329. https://doi.org/10.1016/j.chembiol.2013.12.016

8. CDC. (2022, July 7). *Sleep Difficulties in Adults: United States, 2020.* Www.cdc.gov. https://www.cdc.gov/nchs/products/databriefs/db436.htm

9. Chu, C., Tsuprykov, O., Chen, X., Elitok, S., Krämer, B. K., & Hocher, B. (2021). Relationship Between Vitamin D and Hormones Important for Human Fertility in Reproductive-Aged Women. *Frontiers in endocrinology*, 12, 666687. https://doi.org/10.3389/fendo.2021.666687

10. Coppen, A., & Bolander-Gouaille, C. (2005). "Treatment of depression: time to consider folic acid and vitamin B12." Journal of Psychopharmacology, 19(1), 59-65. https://doi.org/10.1177/0269881105048899

11. Diamanti-Kandarakis, E., Bourguignon, J. P., Giudice, L. C., Hauser, R., Prins, G. S., Soto, A. M., Zoeller, R. T., & Gore, A. C. (2009). Endocrine-disrupting chemicals: An Endocrine Society scientific statement. Endocrine Reviews, 30(4), 293-342. https://doi.org/10.1210/er.2009-0002

12. Fenton, S. E., Ducatman, A., Boobis, A., DeWitt, J. C., Lau, C., Ng, C., Smith, J. S., & Roberts, S. M. (2021). Per- and Polyfluoroalkyl Substance Toxicity and Human Health Review: Current State of Knowledge and Strategies for Informing Future Research. Environmental toxicology and chemistry, 40(3), 606–630. https://doi.org/10.1002/etc.4890

13. Fischer, L. M., da Costa, K. A., Kwock, L., Galanko, J., & Zeisel, S. H. (2010). Dietary choline requirements of women: effects of estrogen and genetic variation. *The American journal of clinical nutrition*, 92(5), 1113–1119. https://doi.org/10.3945/ajcn.2010.30064

14. Gerber, M., Imboden, C., Beck, J., Brand, S., Colledge, F., Eckert, A., Holsboer-Trachsler, E., Pühse, U., & Hatzinger, M. (2020). Effects of Aerobic Exercise on Cortisol Stress Reactivity in Response to the Trier

Social Stress Test in Inpatients with Major Depressive Disorders: A Randomized Controlled Trial. *Journal of clinical medicine, 9*(5), 1419. https://doi.org/10.3390/jcm9051419

15. He, S., Li, H., Yu, Z., Zhang, F., Liang, S., Liu, H., Chen, H., & Lü, M. (2021). The Gut Microbiome and Sex Hormone-Related Diseases. *Frontiers in microbiology, 12*, 711137. https://doi.org/10.3389/fmicb.2021.711137

16. Hendrick, V., Altshuler, L. L., & Suri, R. (1998). Hormonal changes in the postpartum and implications for postpartum depression. *Psychosomatics, 39*(2), 93–101. https://doi.org/10.1016/S0033-3182(98)71355-6

17. Hibbeln, J. R., Linnoila, M., Umhau, J. C., Rawlings, R., George, D. T., & Salem, N., Jr (1998). Essential fatty acids predict metabolites of serotonin and dopamine in cerebrospinal fluid among healthy control subjects, and early- and late-onset alcoholics. *Biological psychiatry, 44*(4), 235–242. https://doi.org/10.1016/s0006-3223(98)00141-3

18. Holick, M. F., & Chen, T. C. (2008). Vitamin D deficiency: a worldwide problem with health consequences. *The American journal of clinical nutrition, 87*(4), 1080S–6S. https://doi.org/10.1093/ajcn/87.4.1080S

19. Kapper, C., Oppelt, P., Ganhör, C., Gyunesh, A. A., Arbeithuber, B., Stelzl, P., & Rezk-Füreder, M. (2024). Minerals and the Menstrual Cycle: Impacts on Ovulation and Endometrial Health. *Nutrients, 16*(7), 1008. https://doi.org/10.3390/nu16071008

20. Kiecolt-Glaser, J. K., Belury, M. A., Andridge, R., Malarkey, W. B., & Glaser, R. (2011). Omega-3 supplementation lowers inflammation and anxiety in medical students: a randomized controlled trial. *Brain, behavior, and immunity, 25*(8), 1725–1734. https://doi.org/10.1016/j.bbi.2011.07.229

21. Kim, K., Mills, J. L., Michels, K. A., Chaljub, E. N., Wactawski-Wende, J., Plowden, T. C., & Mumford, S. L. (2020). Dietary Intakes of Vitamin B-2 (Riboflavin), Vitamin B-6, and Vitamin B-12 and Ovarian Cycle Function among Premenopausal Women. *Journal of the Academy of Nutrition and Dietetics, 120*(5), 885–892. https://doi.org/10.1016/j.jand.2019.10.013

22. Lewinski A.,Brzozowska M., Female infertility as a result of stress-

related hormonal changes, *GREM Gynecological and Reproductive Endocrinology & Metabolism* (2023); Volume 3 - 2/2022:094-098 doi: 10.53260/grem.22302035

23. Long, S. J., & Benton, D. (2013). Effects of vitamin and mineral supplementation on stress, mild psychiatric symptoms, and mood in nonclinical samples: a meta-analysis. *Psychosomatic medicine*, 75(2), 144–153. https://doi.org/10.1097/PSY.0b013e31827d5fbd

24. Mair, K. M., Gaw, R., & MacLean, M. R. (2020). Obesity, estrogens and adipose tissue dysfunction - implications for pulmonary arterial hypertension. Pulmonary circulation, 10(3), 2045894020952019. https://doi.org/10.1177/2045894020952023

25. Mangesi, L., & Zakarija-Grkovic, I. (2016). Treatments for breast engorgement during lactation. *The Cochrane database of systematic reviews*, 2016(6), CD006946. https://doi.org/10.1002/14651858.CD006946.pub3

26. Maniaci, A., Via, L. L., Lentini, M., Pecorino, B., Chiofalo, B., Scibilia, G., Lavalle, S., Luca, A., & Scollo, P. (2025). The Interplay Between Sleep Apnea and Postpartum Depression. *Neurology International*, 17(2), 20–20. https://doi.org/10.3390/neurolint17020020

27. Mazza, E., Troiano, E., Ferro, Y., Lisso, F., Tosi, M., Turco, E., Pujia, R., & Montalcini, T. (2024). Obesity, Dietary Patterns, and Hormonal Balance Modulation: Gender-Specific Impacts. *Nutrients*, 16(11), 1629. https://doi.org/10.3390/nu16111629

28. Moon, J., & Koh, G. (2020). Clinical Evidence and Mechanisms of High-Protein Diet-Induced Weight Loss. *Journal of Obesity & Metabolic Syndrome*, 29(3), 166–173. https://doi.org/10.7570/jomes20028

29. Mostofsky, E., Buring, J.E., Come, S.E. et al. Effect of daily alcohol intake on sex hormone levels among postmenopausal breast cancer survivors on aromatase inhibitor therapy: a randomized controlled crossover pilot study. *Breast Cancer Res* **27**, 5 (2025). https://doi.org/10.1186/s13058-024-01940-4

30. Porri, D., Biesalski, H. K., Limitone, A., Bertuzzo, L., & Cena, H. (2021). Effect of Magnesium Supplementation on women's Health and well-

being. *NFS Journal, 23*, 30-36. https://doi.org/10.1016/j.nfs.2021.03.003
31. Qi, X., Yun, C., Pang, Y., & Qiao, J. (2021). The impact of the gut microbiota on the reproductive and metabolic endocrine system. *Gut microbes, 13*(1), 1-21. https://doi.org/10.1080/19490976.2021.1894070
32. Rahman, M. S., Hossain, K. S., Das, S., Kundu, S., Adegoke, E. O., Rahman, M. A., Hannan, M. A., Uddin, M. J., & Pang, M. G. (2021). Role of Insulin in Health and Disease: An Update. *International journal of molecular sciences, 22*(12), 6403. https://doi.org/10.3390/ijms22126403
33. Rhyu, J., & Yu, R. (2021). Newly discovered endocrine functions of the liver. World journal of hepatology, 13(11), 1611-1628. https://doi.org/10.4254/wjh.v13.i11.1611
34. Rupp, H. A., James, T. W., Ketterson, E. D., Sengelaub, D. R., Ditzen, B., & Heiman, J. R. (2013). Lower sexual interest in postpartum women: relationship to amygdala activation and intranasal oxytocin. *Hormones and behavior, 63*(1), 114-121. https://doi.org/10.1016/j.yhbeh.2012.10.007
35. Schiller, C. E., Meltzer-Brody, S., & Rubinow, D. R. (2015). The role of reproductive hormones in postpartum depression. *CNS spectrums, 20*(1), 48-59. https://doi.org/10.1017/S1092852914000480
36. Sharma, K., Akre, S., Chakole, S., & Wanjari, M. B. (2022). Stress-Induced Diabetes: A Review. *Cureus, 14*(9), e29142. https://doi.org/10.7759/cureus.29142
37. Shobeiri, F., Araste, F. E., Ebrahimi, R., Jenabi, E., & Nazari, M. (2017). Effect of calcium on premenstrual syndrome: A double-blind randomized clinical trial. *Obstetrics & gynecology science, 60*(1), 100-105. https://doi.org/10.5468/ogs.2017.60.1.100
38. Thurston, R. C., Luther, J. F., Wisniewski, S. R., Eng, H., & Wisner, K. L. (2013). Prospective evaluation of nighttime hot flashes during pregnancy and postpartum. *Fertility and sterility, 100*(6), 1667-1672. https://doi.org/10.1016/j.fertnstert.2013.08.020
39. Uvnäs Moberg, K., Ekström-Bergström, A., Buckley, S., Massarotti, C., Pajalic, Z., Luegmair, K., Kotlowska, A., Lengler, L., Olza, I., Grylka-Baeschlin, S., Leahy-Warren, P., Hadjigeorgiu, E., Villarmea,

S., & Dencker, A. (2020). Maternal plasma levels of oxytocin during breastfeeding-A systematic review. *PloS one*, 15(8), e0235806. https://doi.org/10.1371/journal.pone.0235806

40. Ventura, M., Melo, M., & Carrilho, F. (2017). Selenium and Thyroid Disease: From Pathophysiology to Treatment. *International journal of endocrinology*, 2017, 1297658. https://doi.org/10.1155/2017/129765
41. Wilborn, C. D., Kerksick, C. M., Campbell, B. I., Taylor, L. W., Marcello, B. M., Rasmussen, C. J., Greenwood, M. C., Almada, A., & Kreider, R. B. (2004). Effects of Zinc Magnesium Aspartate (ZMA) Supplementation on Training Adaptations and Markers of Anabolism and Catabolism. *Journal of the International Society of Sports Nutrition*, 1(2), 12–20. https://doi.org/10.1186/1550-2783-1-2-12
42. Zheng, YF., Guo, YM., Song, CJ. et al. A cross-sectional study on the relationship between dietary fiber and endometriosis risk based on NHANES 1999–2006. *Sci Rep* 14, 28502 (2024). https://doi.org/10.1038/s41598-024-79746-9

Balancing Hormones Beyond Postpartum

1. Alexander, E. K., Pearce, E. N., Brent, G. A., Brown, R. S., Chen, H., Dosiou, C., & Sullivan, S. (2017). Guidelines of the American Thyroid Association for the diagnosis and management of thyroid disease during pregnancy and the postpartum. *Thyroid*, 27(3), 315-389. https://doi.org/10.1089/thy.2016.0457
2. Alur-Gupta, S., Boland, M. R., Barnhart, K. T., Sammel, M. D., & Dokras, A. (2021). Postpartum complications increased in women with polycystic ovary syndrome. *American journal of obstetrics and gynecology*, 224(3), 280.e1–280.e13. https://doi.org/10.1016/j.ajog.2020.08.048
3. Basnet, J., Eissa, M. A., Yanes Cardozo, L. L., Romero, D. G., & Rezq, S. (2024). Impact of Probiotics and Prebiotics on Gut Microbiome and Hormonal Regulation. *Gastrointestinal Disorders*, 6(4), 801-815. https://doi.org/10.3390/gidisord6040056

4. Buck Louis, G. M., Gray, L. E., Marcus, M., Ojeda, S. R., Pescovitz, O. H., Witchel, S. F., ... & Bourguignon, J. P. (2016). Environmental factors and puberty timing: Expert panel research needs. Pediatrics, 121(Supplement 3), S192-S207. https://doi.org/10.1542/peds.2007-1813D
5. CDC. (2022, July 7). Sleep Difficulties in Adults: United States, 2020. Www.cdc.gov. https://www.cdc.gov/nchs/products/databriefs/db436.htm
6. Centers for Disease Control and Prevention. (2022). Polycystic ovary syndrome (PCOS). Retrieved from https://www.cdc.gov/diabetes/risk-factors/pcos-polycystic-ovary-syndrome.html
7. Chrousos, G. P. (2009). "Stress and disorders of the stress system." Nature Reviews Endocrinology, 5(7), 374-381. https://doi.org/10.1038/nrendo.2009.106
8. Chu B, Marwaha K, Sanvictores T, et al. Physiology, Stress Reaction. [Updated 2024 May 7]. In: StatPearls [Internet]. Treasure Island (FL): StatPearls Publishing; 2025 Jan-. Available from: https://www.ncbi.nlm.nih.gov/books/NBK541120/
9. Cleary, M. P., & Grossmann, M. E. (2009). Minireview: Obesity and breast cancer: the estrogen connection. Endocrinology, 150(6), 2537–2542. https://doi.org/10.1210/en.2009-0070
10. De Nys, L., Anderson, K., Ofosu, E. F., Ryde, G. C., Connelly, J., & Whittaker, A. C. (2022). The effects of physical activity on cortisol and sleep: A systematic review and meta-analysis. Psychoneuroendocrinology, 143(143), 105843. https://doi.org/10.1016/j.psyneuen.2022.105843
11. Diamanti-Kandarakis, E., Bourguignon, J. P., Giudice, L. C., Hauser, R., Prins, G. S., Soto, A. M., ... & Gore, A. C. (2009). Endocrine-disrupting chemicals: An Endocrine Society scientific statement. Endocrine Reviews, 30(4), 293–342. https://doi.org/10.1210/er.2009-0002
12. Fowke, J. H., Longcope, C., & Hebert, J. R. (2000). Brassica vegetable consumption shifts estrogen metabolism in healthy postmenopausal women. Cancer epidemiology, biomarkers & prevention: a publication of the American Association for Cancer Research, cosponsored by the

American Society of Preventive Oncology, 9(8), 773–779.
13. Gaskins, A. J., Mumford, S. L., Zhang, C., Wactawski-Wende, J., Hovey, K. M., Whitcomb, B. W., Howards, P. P., Perkins, N. J., Yeung, E., Schisterman, E. F., & BioCycle Study Group (2009). Effect of daily fiber intake on reproductive function: the BioCycle Study. The American journal of clinical nutrition, 90(4), 1061–1069. https://doi.org/10.3945/ajcn.2009.27990
14. Gore, A. C., Chappell, V. A., Fenton, S. E., Flaws, J. A., Nadal, A., Prins, G. S., & Zoeller, R. T. (2015). EDC-2: The Endocrine Society's second scientific statement on endocrine-disrupting chemicals. Endocrine Reviews, 36(6), E1-E150. https://doi.org/10.1210/er.2015-1010
15. Holst, J. P., Soldin, O. P., Guo, T., & Soldin, S. J. (2004). Steroid hormones: relevance and measurement in the clinical laboratory. Clinics in laboratory medicine, 24(1), 105–118. https://doi.org/10.1016/j.cll.2004.01.004
16. Kamaly, H. F., & Sharkawy, A. A. (2023). Hormonal residues in chicken and cattle meat: A risk threat the present and future consumer health. Food and Chemical Toxicology, 182, 114172. https://doi.org/10.1016/j.fct.2023.114172
17. Karaivanova, T., Yaneva, E., Dimitrova, K., & Ilieva, A. (2020). Hormonal dynamics during the postpartum period: Clinical implications and recommendations. Endocrine Disorders Review, 12(4), 45-58. https://doi.org/10.1016/edr.2020.06.002
18. Kasarinaite, A., Sinton, M., Saunders, P. T. K., & Hay, D. C. (2023). The Influence of Sex Hormones in Liver Function and Disease. Cells, 12(12), 1604. https://doi.org/10.3390/cells12121604Bhardwaj, P., Au, C. C., Benito-Martin, A., Ladumor, H., Oshchepkova, S., Moges, R., & Brown, K. A. (2019). Estrogens and breast cancer: Mechanisms involved in obesity-related development, growth and progression. The Journal of steroid biochemistry and molecular biology, 189, 161–170. https://doi.org/10.1016/j.jsbmb.2019.03.002
19. Köhrle J. (2023). Selenium, Iodine and Iron-Essential Trace Elements for Thyroid Hormone Synthesis and Metabolism. International journal

of molecular sciences, 24(4), 3393. https://doi.org/10.3390/ijms24043393
20. Levine, H., Jørgensen, N., Martino-Andrade, A., Mendiola, J., Weksler-Derri, D., Mindlis, I., ... & Swan, S. H. (2017). Temporal trends in sperm count: A systematic review and meta-regression analysis. Human Reproduction Update, 23(6), 646–659. https://doi.org/10.1093/humupd/dmx022
21. Mair, K. M., Gaw, R., & MacLean, M. R. (2020). Obesity, estrogens and adipose tissue dysfunction - implications for pulmonary arterial hypertension. Pulmonary circulation, 10(3), 2045894020952019. https://doi.org/10.1177/2045894020952023
22. Malekinejad, H., & Rezabakhsh, A. (2015). Hormones in Dairy Foods and Their Impact on Public Health - A Narrative Review Article. Iranian journal of public health, 44(6), 742–758.
23. Marlatt, V. L., Bayen, S., Castaneda-Cortès, D., Delbès, G., Grigorova, P., Langlois, V. S., Martyniuk, C. J., Metcalfe, C. D., Parent, L., Rwigemera, A., Thomson, P., & Van Der Kraak, G. (2022). Impacts of endocrine disrupting chemicals on reproduction in wildlife and humans. Environmental Research, 208, 112584. https://doi.org/10.1016/j.envres.2021.112584
24. Mazza, E., Troiano, E., Ferro, Y., Fabrizia Lisso, Tosi, M., Turco, E., Pujia, R., & Tiziana Montalcini. (2024). Obesity, Dietary Patterns, and Hormonal Balance Modulation: Gender-Specific Impacts. Nutrients, 16(11), 1629–1629. https://doi.org/10.3390/nu16111629
25. National Institute of Environmental Health Sciences. (2024, July 22). Endocrine Disruptors. National Institute of Environmental Health Sciences. https://www.niehs.nih.gov/health/topics/agents/endocrine
26. Rhyu, J., & Yu, R. (2021). Newly discovered endocrine functions of the liver. World journal of hepatology, 13(11), 1611–1628. https://doi.org/10.4254/wjh.v13.i11.161
27. Volk, K. M., Pogrebna, V. V., Roberts, J. A., Zachry, J. E., Blythe, S. N., & Toporikova, N. (2017). High-Fat, High-Sugar Diet Disrupts the Preovulatory Hormone Surge and Induces Cystic Ovaries in Cycling Female Rats. Journal of the Endocrine Society, 1(12), 1488–1505.

https://doi.org/10.1210/js.2017-00305
28. Zhao, H., Gui, W., Liu, S., Zhao, F., Fan, W., Jing, F., & Sun, C. (2024). Ultra-processed foods intake and sex hormone levels among children and adolescents aged 6-19 years: a cross-sectional study. Frontiers in nutrition, 11, 1451481. https://doi.org/10.3389/fnut.2024.1451481

Gut Health Restoration

1. Aguirre-Cruz, G., León-López, A., Cruz-Gómez, V., Jiménez-Alvarado, R., & Aguirre-Álvarez, G. (2020). Collagen Hydrolysates for Skin Protection: Oral Administration and Topical Formulation. Antioxidants (Basel, Switzerland), 9(2), 181. https://doi.org/10.3390/antiox9020181
2. Anderson, J. W., Allgood, L. D., Lawrence, A., Altringer, L. A., Jerdack, G. R., Hengehold, D. A., & Morel, J. G. (2000). Cholesterol-lowering effects of psyllium intake adjunctive to diet therapy in men and women with hypercholesterolemia: Meta-analysis of 8 controlled trials. American Journal of Clinical Nutrition, 71(2), 472–479. https://doi.org/10.1093/ajcn/71.2.472
3. Anderson, J. W., Baird, P., Davis, R. H., Ferreri, S., Knudtson, M., Koraym, A., ... & Williams, C. L. (2009). Health benefits of dietary fiber. Nutrition Reviews, 67(4), 188-205. https://doi.org/10.1111/j.1753-4887.2009.00189.x
4. Ankri, S., & Mirelman, D. (1999). Antimicrobial properties of allicin from garlic. Microbes and Infection, 1(2), 125–129. https://doi.org/10.1016/s1286-4579(99)80003-3
5. Belkaid, Y., & Hand, T. W. (2014). Role of the microbiota in immunity and inflammation. Cell, 157(1), 121–141. https://doi.org/10.1016/j.cell.2014.03.011
6. Boudreau, M. D., Olson, G. R., Tryndyak, V. P., Bryant, M. S., Felton, R. P., & Beland, F. A. (2017). From the Cover: Aloin, a Component of the Aloe Vera Plant Leaf, Induces Pathological Changes and Modulates the Composition of Microbiota in the Large Intestines of F344/N Male Rats. Toxicological Sciences, 158(2), 302–318. https://doi.org/10.1093/

toxsci/kfx105
7. Bressa, C., Bailén-Andrino, M., Pérez-Santiago, J., González-Soltero, R., Pérez, M., Montalvo-Lominchar, M. G., ... & Moreno, D. (2017). Differences in gut microbiota profile between women with active lifestyle and sedentary women. PLoS ONE, 12(2), e0171352. https://doi.org/10.1371/journal.pone.0171352
8. Calder, P.C., Yaqoob, P. Glutamine and the immune system. Amino Acids 17, 227–241 (1999). https://doi.org/10.1007/BF01366922
9. Canfora, E. E., Meex, R. C. R., Venema, K., & Blaak, E. E. (2019). Gut microbial metabolites in obesity, NAFLD and T2DM. Nature Reviews Endocrinology, 15(5), 261-273. https://doi.org/10.1038/s41574-019-0156-z
10. Claesson, M. J., Jeffery, I. B., Conde, S., Power, S. E., O'Connor, E. M., Cusack, S., ... & O'Toole, P. W. (2011). Gut microbiota composition correlates with diet and health in the elderly. Nature, 488(7410), 178–184. https://doi.org/10.1038/nature11319
11. Clark, K. L., Sebastianelli, W., Flechsenhar, K. R., Aukermann, D., Meza, F., Millard, R. L., ... & Deitch, J. R. (2008). 24-week study on the use of collagen hydrolysate as a dietary supplement in athletes with activity-related joint pain. Current Medical Research and Opinion, 24(5), 1485–1496. https://doi.org/10.1185/030079908X291967
12. Clarke, G., Grenham, S., Scully, P., Fitzgerald, P., Moloney, R. D., Shanahan, F., Dinan, T. G., & Cryan, J. F. (2013). The microbiome-gut-brain axis during early life regulates the hippocampal serotonergic system in a sex-dependent manner. Molecular psychiatry, 18(6), 666–673. https://doi.org/10.1038/mp.2012.77
13. Clemente, J. C., Ursell, L. K., Parfrey, L. W., & Knight, R. (2012). The impact of the gut microbiota on human health: an integrative view. Cell, 148(6), 1258–1270. https://doi.org/10.1016/j.cell.2012.01.035
14. Corrie, L., Awasthi, A., Kaur, J., Vishwas, S., Gulati, M., Kaur, I. P., Gupta, G., Kommineni, N., Dua, K., & Singh, S. K. (2023). Interplay of Gut Microbiota in Polycystic Ovarian Syndrome: Role of Gut Microbiota, Mechanistic Pathways and Potential Treatment Strategies. Pharmaceu-

ticals (Basel, Switzerland), 16(2), 197. https://doi.org/10.3390/ph16020197

15. Cronin, P., Joyce, S. A., O'Toole, P. W., & O'Connor, E. M. (2021). Dietary Fibre Modulates the Gut Microbiota. Nutrients, 13(5), 1655. https://doi.org/10.3390/nu13051655

16. Cruzat, V., Macedo Rogero, M., Noel Keane, K., Curi, R., & Newsholme, P. (2018). Glutamine: Metabolism and Immune Function, Supplementation and Clinical Translation. Nutrients, 10(11), 1564. https://doi.org/10.3390/nu10111564

17. Cryan, J. F., O'Riordan, K. J., Cowan, C. S. M., Sandhu, K. V., Bastiaanssen, T. F. S., Boehme, M., ... & Dinan, T. G. (2019). The microbiota-gut-brain axis. Physiological Reviews, 99(4), 1877-2013. https://doi.org/10.1152/physrev.00018.2018

18. Czerucka, D., Piche, T., & Rampal, P. (2007). Review article: yeast as probiotics – Saccharomyces boulardii. Alimentary Pharmacology & Therapeutics, 26(6), 767–778. https://doi.org/10.1111/j.1365-2036.2007.03442.x

19. Deters, B. J., & Saleem, M. (2021). The role of glutamine in supporting gut health and neuropsychiatric factors. Food Science and Human Wellness, 10(2), 149–154. https://doi.org/10.1016/j.fshw.2021.02.003

20. Dethlefsen, L., & Relman, D. A. (2011). Incomplete recovery and individualized responses of the human distal gut microbiota to repeated antibiotic perturbation. Proceedings of the National Academy of Sciences, 108(Supplement 1), 4554-4561. https://doi.org/10.1073/pnas.1000087107

21. Dinan, T. G., Stanton, C., & Cryan, J. F. (2013). Psychobiotics: a novel class of psychotropic. Biological psychiatry, 74(10), 720–726. https://doi.org/10.1016/j.biopsych.2013.05.001

22. Dominguez-Bello, M. G., Costello, E. K., Contreras, M., Magris, M., Hidalgo, G., & et al. (2010). Delivery mode shapes the acquisition and structure of the initial microbiota across multiple body habitats in newborns. Proceedings of the National Academy of Sciences, 107(26), 11971-11975.

23. Efthymakis, K., & Neri, M. (2022). The role of Zinc L-Carnosine in the prevention and treatment of gastrointestinal mucosal disease in humans: a review. Clinics and Research in Hepatology and Gastroenterology, 46(7), 101954. https://doi.org/10.1016/j.clinre.2022.101954
24. Flores, R., Caporaso, J. G., & Knight, R. (2022). The role of the human microbiome in regulating metabolism. Trends in Endocrinology & Metabolism, 33(10), 703-715.
25. Food and Drug Administration. (2006). Health claim notification for whole grain foods. U.S. Department of Health and Human Services. Retrieved from https://www.fda.gov/food/nutrition-food-labeling-and-critical-foods/health-claim-notification-whole-grain-foods
26. Foster, J. A., Rinaman, L., & Cryan, J. F. (2017). Stress & the gut-brain axis: Regulation by the microbiome. Neurobiology of stress, 7, 124–136. https://doi.org/10.1016/j.ynstr.2017.03.001
27. Franzosa, E. A., Sirota-Madi, A., Avila-Pacheco, J., Fornelos, N., Haiser, H. J., Reinker, S., ... & Huttenhower, C. (2019). Gut microbiome structure and metabolic activity in inflammatory bowel disease. Nature Microbiology, 4(2), 293-305. https://doi.org/10.1038/s41564-018-0306-4
28. Fu, J., Zheng, Y., Gao, Y., & Xu, W. (2022). Dietary Fiber Intake and Gut Microbiota in Human Health. Microorganisms, 10(12), 2507. https://doi.org/10.3390/microorganisms10122507
29. Geng, J., Ni, Q., Sun, W., Li, L., & Feng, X. (2022). The links between gut microbiota and obesity and obesity related diseases. Biomedicine & Pharmacotherapy, 147, 112678. https://doi.org/10.1016/j.biopha.2022.112678
30. Ghosh, T. S., Shanahan, F., & O'Toole, P. W. (2022). The gut microbiome as a modulator of healthy ageing. Nature reviews. Gastroenterology & hepatology, 19(9), 565–584. https://doi.org/10.1038/s41575-022-00605-x
31. Gibson, G. R., Probert, H. M., Loo, J. V., Rastall, R. A., & Roberfroid, M. B. (2004). Dietary modulation of the human colonic microbiota: updating the concept of prebiotics. Nutrition research reviews, 17(2), 259–275. https://doi.org/10.1079/NRR200479

32. Gill, P. A., Inniss, S., Kumagai, T., Rahman, F. Z., & Smith, A. M. (2022). The Role of Diet and Gut Microbiota in Regulating Gastrointestinal and Inflammatory Disease. Frontiers in immunology, 13, 866059. https://doi.org/10.3389/fimmu.2022.866059
33. Hassan, N. E., El-Masry, S. A., El Shebini, S. M., Ahmed, N. H., Mehanna, N. S., Abdel Wahed, M. M., Amine, D., Hashish, A., Selim, M., Afify, M. A. S., & Alian, K. (2024). Effect of weight loss program using prebiotics and probiotics on body composition, physique, and metabolic products: longitudinal intervention study. Scientific reports, 14(1), 10960. https://doi.org/10.1038/s41598-024-61130-2
34. Heyman, M. B. (2006). Lactose intolerance in infants, children, and adolescents. Pediatrics, 118(3), 1279–1286. https://doi.org/10.1542/peds.2006-1721
35. Hill, C., Guarner, F., Reid, G., Gibson, G. R., Merenstein, D. J., Pot, B., ... & Sanders, M. E. (2014). The International Scientific Association for Probiotics and Prebiotics consensus statement on the scope and appropriate use of the term probiotic. Nature Reviews Gastroenterology & Hepatology, 11(8), 506-514. https://doi.org/10.1038/nrgastro.2014.66
36. Hill, C., Guarner, F., Reid, G., Gibson, G. R., Merenstein, D. J., Pot, B., ... & Sanders, M. E. (2014). The International Scientific Association for Probiotics and Prebiotics consensus statement on the scope and appropriate use of the term probiotic. Nature Reviews Gastroenterology & Hepatology, 11(8), 506-514. https://doi.org/10.1038/nrgastro.2014.66
37. Hill, C., Guarner, F., Reid, G., Gibson, G. R., Merenstein, D. J., Pot, B., Morelli, L., Canani, R. B., Flint, H. J., Salminen, S., Calder, P. C., & Sanders, M. E. (2014). The International Scientific Association for Probiotics and Prebiotics consensus statement on the scope and appropriate use of the term probiotic. Nature Reviews Gastroenterology & Hepatology, 11(8), 506–514. https://doi.org/10.1038/nrgastro.2014.66
38. Ianiro, G., Pecere, S., Giorgio, V., Gasbarrini, A., & Cammarota, G. (2016). Digestive Enzyme Supplementation in Gastrointestinal Diseases.

Current drug metabolism, 17(2), 187–193. https://doi.org/10.2174/1389200021702160114150137

39. Jadhav, H. B., & Annapure, U. S. (2023). Triglycerides of medium-chain fatty acids: a concise review. Journal of food science and technology, 60(8), 2143–2152. https://doi.org/10.1007/s13197-022-05499-w

40. Jia, L., Wu, J., Lei, Y., Kong, F., Zhang, R., Sun, J., Wang, L., Li, Z., Shi, J., Wang, Y., Wei, Y., Zhang, K., & Lei, Z. (2022). Oregano Essential Oils Mediated Intestinal Microbiota and Metabolites and Improved Growth Performance and Intestinal Barrier Function in Sheep. Frontiers in immunology, 13, 908015. https://doi.org/10.3389/fimmu.2022.908015

41. Jovanovski, E., Yashpal, S., Komishon, A., Zurbau, A., Blanco Mejia, S., Ho, H. V. T., Li, D., Sievenpiper, J., Duvnjak, L., & Vuksan, V. (2018). Effect of psyllium (Plantago ovata) fiber on LDL cholesterol and alternative lipid targets, non-HDL cholesterol and apolipoprotein B: a systematic review and meta-analysis of randomized controlled trials. The American journal of clinical nutrition, 108(5), 922–932. https://doi.org/10.1093/ajcn/nqy115

42. Kelesidis, T., & Pothoulakis, C. (2012). Efficacy and safety of the probiotic Saccharomyces boulardii for the prevention and therapy of gastrointestinal disorders. Therapeutic Advances in Gastroenterology, 5(2), 111–125. https://doi.org/10.1177/1756283X11428502

43. Kim, Y. S., Unno, T., Kim, B. Y., & Park, M. S. (2020). Sex Differences in Gut Microbiota. The world journal of men's health, 38(1), 48–60. https://doi.org/10.5534/wjmh.190009

44. Koren, O., Goodrich, J. K., Cullender, T. C., Spor, A., Laitinen, K., Backhed, H. K., ... & Ley, R. E. (2012). Host remodeling of the gut microbiome and metabolic changes during pregnancy. Cell, 150(3), 470–480. https://doi.org/10.1016/j.cell.2012.07.008

45. Kumari, N., Kumari, R., Dua, A., Singh, M., Kumar, R., Singh, P., Duyar-Ayerdi, S., Pradeep, S., Ojesina, A. I., & Kumar, R. (2024). From Gut to Hormones: Unraveling the Role of Gut Microbiota in (Phyto)Estrogen Modulation in Health and Disease. Molecular nutrition & food research, 68(6), e2300688. https://doi.org/10.1002/mnfr.202300688

46. Kumari, N., Kumari, R., Dua, A., Singh, M., Kumar, R., Singh, P., Duyar-Ayerdi, S., Pradeep, S., Ojesina, A. I., & Kumar, R. (2024). From Gut to Hormones: Unraveling the Role of Gut Microbiota in (Phyto)Estrogen Modulation in Health and Disease. Molecular nutrition & food research, 68(6), e2300688

47. Langmead, L., & Rampton, D. S. (2001). Review article: herbal treatment in gastrointestinal and liver disease—benefits and dangers. Alimentary pharmacology & therapeutics, 15(9), 1239–1252. https://doi.org/10.1046/j.1365-2036.2001.01053.x

48. Langmead, L., Feakins, R. M., Goldthorpe, S., & Rampton, D. S. (2004). Randomized, double-blind, placebo-controlled trial of oral aloe vera gel for active ulcerative colitis. Alimentary Pharmacology & Therapeutics, 19(7), 739–747. https://doi.org/10.1111/j.1365-2036.2004.01902.x

49. Langmead, L., Feakins, R. M., Goldthorpe, S., Holt, H., Tsironi, E., De Silva, A., Jewell, D. P., & Rampton, D. S. (2004). Randomized, double-blind, placebo-controlled trial of oral aloe vera gel for active ulcerative colitis. Alimentary pharmacology & therapeutics, 19(7), 739–747. https://doi.org/10.1111/j.1365-2036.2004.01902.x

50. Le Phan, T. H., Park, S. Y., Jung, H. J., Kim, M. W., Cho, E., Shim, K. S., Shin, E., Yoon, J. H., Maeng, H. J., Kang, J. H., & Oh, S. H. (2021). The Role of Processed Aloe vera Gel in Intestinal Tight Junction: An In Vivo and In Vitro Study. International journal of molecular sciences, 22(12), 6515. https://doi.org/10.3390/ijms22126515

51. Looijer-van Langen, M. A., & Dieleman, L. A. (2009). Prebiotics in chronic intestinal inflammation. Inflammatory bowel diseases, 15(3), 454–462. https://doi.org/10.1002/ibd.20737

52. Lowe M. E. (1994). Pancreatic triglyceride lipase and colipase: insights into dietary fat digestion. Gastroenterology, 107(5), 1524–1536. https://doi.org/10.1016/0016-5085(94)90559-2

53. Madison, A., & Kiecolt-Glaser, J. K. (2019). Stress, depression, diet, and the gut microbiota: human-bacteria interactions at the core of psychoneuroimmunology and nutrition. Current opinion in behavioral sciences, 28, 105–110. https://doi.org/10.1016/j.cobeha.2019.01.011

54. Mahmood, A., FitzGerald, A. J., Marchbank, T., Ntatsaki, E., Murray, D., Ghosh, S., & Playford, R. J. (2007). Zinc carnosine, a health food supplement that stabilises small bowel integrity and stimulates gut repair processes. Gut, 56(2), 168–175. https://doi.org/10.1136/gut.200 6.099929
55. Maria-Nefeli Tsetseri, Silman, A. J., Keene, D., & Dakin, S. G. (2023). The role of the microbiome in rheumatoid arthritis: a review. Rheumatology Advances in Practice, 7(2). https://doi.org/10.1093/rap/rkad034
56. Mariaule, V., Kriaa, A., Soussou, S., Rhimi, S., Boudaya, H., Hernandez, J., Maguin, E., Lesner, A., & Rhimi, M. (2021). Digestive Inflammation: Role of Proteolytic Dysregulation. International journal of molecular sciences, 22(6), 2817. https://doi.org/10.3390/ijms22062817
57. McFarland, L. V. (2010). Systematic review and meta-analysis of Saccharomyces boulardii in adult patients. World Journal of Gastroenterology, 16(18), 2202–2222. https://doi.org/10.3748/wjg.v16.i18.2202
58. McFarland, L. V. (2010). Systematic review and meta-analysis of Saccharomyces boulardii in adult patients. World Journal of Gastroenterology, 16(18), 2202–2222. https://doi.org/10.3748/wjg.v16.i18.2202
59. Montalto, M., Curigliano, V., & Santoro, L. (2006). Management and treatment of lactose malabsorption. World Journal of Gastroenterology, 12(2), 187–191. https://doi.org/10.3748/wjg.v12.i2.187
60. Montenegro, J., Armet, A. M., Willing, B. P., Deehan, E. C., Fassini, P. G., Mota, J. F., Walter, J., & Prado, C. M. (2023). Exploring the Influence of Gut Microbiome on Energy Metabolism in Humans. Advances in nutrition (Bethesda, Md.), 14(4), 840–857. https://doi.org/10.1016/ j.advnut.2023.03.015
61. Nageswaran Sivalingam, Suresh Pichandi, Chapla, A., Dinakaran, A., & Jacob, M. (2011). Zinc protects against indomethacin-induced damage in the rat small intestine. European Journal of Pharmacology, 654(1), 106–116. https://doi.org/10.1016/j.ejphar.2010.12.014
62. Napolitano, M., Fasulo, E., Ungaro, F., Massimino, L., Sinagra, E., Danese, S., & Mandarino, F. V. (2023). Gut Dysbiosis in Irritable Bowel Syndrome: A Narrative Review on Correlation with Disease Subtypes

and Novel Therapeutic Implications. Microorganisms, 11(10), 2369. https://doi.org/10.3390/microorganisms11102369

63. Niu, M., Li, Q., Zhang, J., Wen, F., Dang, W., Duan, G., Li, H., Ruan, W., Yang, P., Guan, C., Tian, H., Gao, X., Zhang, S., Yuan, F., & Han, Y. (2019). Characterization of Intestinal Microbiota and Probiotics Treatment in Children with Autism Spectrum Disorders in China. Frontiers in neurology, 10, 1084. https://doi.org/10.3389/fneur.2019.01084

64. O'Toole, P. W., & Jeffery, I. B. (2015). Gut microbiota and aging. Science, 350(6265), 1214-1215. https://doi.org/10.1126/science.aac8469

65. Ostan, R., Bucci, L., Pini, E., Nikkïla, J., Monti, D., Satokari, R., Franceschi, C., Brigidi, P., & De Vos, W. (2010). Through ageing, and beyond: gut microbiota and inflammatory status in seniors and centenarians. PloS one, 5(5), e10667. https://doi.org/10.1371/journal.pone.0010667

66. Ouwehand, A. C., Salminen, S., & Isolauri, E. (2002). Probiotics: An overview of beneficial effects. Antonie Van Leeuwenhoek, 82(1-4), 279–289. https://doi.org/10.1023/A:1020620607611

67. Pan, R., Wang, L., Xu, X., Chen, Y., Wang, H., Wang, G., Zhao, J., & Chen, W. (2022). Crosstalk between the Gut Microbiome and Colonic Motility in Chronic Constipation: Potential Mechanisms and Microbiota Modulation. Nutrients, 14(18), 3704. https://doi.org/10.3390/nu14183704

68. Parizadeh, M., & Arrieta, M.-C. (2023). The global human gut microbiome: genes, lifestyles, and diet. Trends in Molecular Medicine, 29(10), S1471-4914(23)001521. https://doi.org/10.1016/j.molmed.2023.07.002

69. Pastors, J. G., Blaisdell, P. W., Balm, T. K., Asplin, C. M., & Pohl, S. L. (1991). Psyllium fiber reduces rise in postprandial glucose and insulin concentrations in patients with non-insulin-dependent diabetes. The American journal of clinical nutrition, 53(6), 1431–1435. https://doi.org/10.1093/ajcn/53.6.1431

70. Pedroza Matute, S., & Iyavoo, S. (2023). Exploring the gut microbiota: lifestyle choices, disease associations, and personal genomics. Frontiers in nutrition, 10, 1225120. https://doi.org/10.3389/fnut.2023.1225120

71. Queen, J., Zhang, J., & Sears, C. L. (2020). Oral antibiotic use and chronic disease: long-term health impact beyond antimicrobial resistance and Clostridioides difficile. Gut microbes, 11(4), 1092–1103. https://doi.org/10.1080/19490976.2019.1706425
72. Radha, M. H., & Laxmipriya, N. P. (2015). Evaluation of biological properties and clinical effectiveness of Aloe vera: A systematic review. Journal of Traditional and Complementary Medicine, 5(1), 21–26. https://doi.org/10.1016/j.jtcme.2014.10.006
73. Ried, K., Travica, N., Dorairaj, R., & Sali, A. (2020). Herbal formula improves upper and lower gastrointestinal symptoms and gut health in Australian adults with digestive disorders. Nutrition Research (New York, N.Y.), 76, 37–51. https://doi.org/10.1016/j.nutres.2020.02.008
74. Saboo, B., Misra, A., Kalra, S., Mohan, V., Aravind, S. R., Joshi, S., Chowdhury, S., Sahay, R., Kesavadev, J., John, M., Kapoor, N., Das, S., Krishnan, D., & Salis, S. (2022). Role and importance of high fiber in diabetes management in India. Diabetes & Metabolic Syndrome: Clinical Research & Reviews, 16(5), 102480. https://doi.org/10.1016/j.dsx.2022.102480
75. Sanders, M. E., Guarner, F., Guerrant, R., Holt, P. R., Quigley, E. M. M., Sartor, R. B., Sherman, P. M., & Mayer, E. A. (2013). An update on the use and investigation of probiotics in health and disease. Gut, 62(5), 787–796. https://doi.org/10.1136/gutjnl-2012-302504
76. Schaub, A.-C., Schneider, E., Vazquez-Castellanos, J. F., Schweinfurth, N., Kettelhack, C., Doll, J. P. K., Yamanbaeva, G., Mählmann, L., Brand, S., Beglinger, C., Borgwardt, S., Raes, J., Schmidt, A., & Lang, U. E. (2022). Clinical, gut microbial and neural effects of a probiotic add-on therapy in depressed patients: a randomized controlled trial. Translational Psychiatry, 12(1), 1–10. https://doi.org/10.1038/s41398-022-01977-z
77. Slavin, J. (2013). Fiber and prebiotics: Mechanisms and health benefits. Nutrients, 5(4), 1417-1435. https://doi.org/10.3390/nu5041417
78. Sturniolo, G. C., Di Leo, V., Ferronato, A., D'Odorico, A., & D'Incà, R. (2001). Zinc supplementation tightens "leaky gut" in Crohn's disease. Inflammatory Bowel Diseases, 7(2), 94–98. https://doi.org/10.1097/

00054725-200105000-00003

79. Sun, Y., Gao, S., Ye, C., & Zhao, W. (2023). Gut microbiota dysbiosis in polycystic ovary syndrome: Mechanisms of progression and clinical applications. Frontiers in cellular and infection microbiology, 13, 1142041. https://doi.org/10.3389/fcimb.2023.1142041

80. Tamburini, S., Shen, N., Wu, H. C., & Clemente, J. C. (2016). The microbiome in early life: implications for health outcomes. Nature medicine, 22(7), 713–722. https://doi.org/10.1038/nm.4142

81. Thomas, A., Thomas, A., & Butler-Sanchez, M. (2021). Dietary Modification for the Restoration of Gut Microbiome and Management of Symptoms in Irritable Bowel Syndrome. American journal of lifestyle medicine, 16(5), 608–621. https://doi.org/10.1177/15598276211012968

82. Wang, H., Zhang, H., Gao, Z., Zhang, Q., & Gu, C. (2022). The mechanism of berberine alleviating metabolic disorder based on gut microbiome. Frontiers in cellular and infection microbiology, 12, 854885. https://doi.org/10.3389/fcimb.2022.854885

83. Xie, L., Zhao, H., & Chen, W. (2023). Relationship between gut microbiota and thyroid function: a two-sample Mendelian randomization study. Frontiers in Endocrinology, 14. https://doi.org/10.3389/fendo.2023.1240752

84. Xin, XY., Zhou, J., Liu, GG. et al. Anti-inflammatory activity of collagen peptide in vitro and its effect on improving ulcerative colitis. npj Sci Food 9, 1 (2025). https://doi.org/10.1038/s41538-024-00367-7

85. Yagnik, D., Ward, M., & Shah, A. J. (2021). Antibacterial apple cider vinegar eradicates methicillin resistant Staphylococcus aureus and resistant Escherichia coli. Scientific reports, 11(1), 1854. https://doi.org/10.1038/s41598-020-78407-xCamilleri, M., & Vella, A. (2022). What to do about the leaky gut. Gut, 71(2), 424–435. https://doi.org/10.1136/gutjnl-2021-325428

86. Yang, C., Liu, S., Li, H., Bai, X., Shan, S., Gao, P., & Dong, X. (2021). The effects of psyllium husk on gut microbiota composition and function in chronically constipated women of reproductive age using 16S rRNA gene sequencing analysis. Aging, 13(11), 15366–15383. https://doi.org/

10.18632/aging.203095

87. Zdzieblik, D., Oesser, S., Gollhofer, A., König, D., & Schwarz, R. (2015). Collagen peptide supplementation in combination with resistance training improves body composition and increases muscle strength in elderly sarcopenic men: A randomized controlled trial. British Journal of Nutrition, 114(8), 1237–1245. https://doi.org/10.1017/S0007114515002810
88. Zhu, Q., Chen, B., Zhang, F., Zhang, B., Guo, Y., Pang, M., Huang, L., & Wang, T. (2024). Toxic and essential metals: metabolic interactions with the gut microbiota and health implications. Frontiers in Nutrition, 11. https://doi.org/10.3389/fnut.2024.1448388

Strategies for Sleep Struggles

1. Baattaiah, B.A., Alharbi, M.D., Babteen, N.M. et al. The relationship between fatigue, sleep quality, resilience, and the risk of postpartum depression: an emphasis on maternal mental health. BMC Psychol 11, 10 (2023). https://doi.org/10.1186/s40359-023-01043-3
2. Bent, S., Padula, A., Moore, D., Patterson, M., & Mehling, W. (2006). Valerian for sleep: a systematic review and meta-analysis. The American journal of medicine, 119(12), 1005–1012. https://doi.org/10.1016/j.amjmed.2006.02.026
3. Bhaskar, S., Hemavathy, D., & Prasad, S. (2016). Prevalence of chronic insomnia in adult patients and its correlation with medical comorbidities. Journal of family medicine and primary care, 5(4), 780–784. https://doi.org/10.4103/2249-4863.201153
4. Byrne, E. (2019). The relationship between insomnia and complex diseases—insights from genetic data. Genome Medicine, 11(1). https://doi.org/10.1186/s13073-019-0668-0
5. Costello, R.B., Lentino, C.V., Boyd, C.C. et al. The effectiveness of melatonin for promoting healthy sleep: a rapid evidence assessment of the literature. Nutr J 13, 106 (2014). https://doi.org/10.1186/1475-2891-13-106Kim, M., Seol, J., Sato, T., Fukamizu, Y., Sakurai, T., & Okura,

T. (2022). Effect of 12-Week Intake of Nicotinamide Mononucleotide on Sleep Quality, Fatigue, and Physical Performance in Older Japanese Adults: A Randomized, Double-Blind Placebo-Controlled Study. Nutrients, 14(4), 755. https://doi.org/10.3390/nu14040755

6. Gueron-Sela, N., Shahar, G., Volkovich, E., & Tikotzky, L. (2021). Prenatal maternal sleep and trajectories of postpartum depression and anxiety symptoms. Journal of sleep research, 30(4), e13258. https://doi.org/10.1111/jsr.13258

7. Gupta, S., Shankar, E., & Srivastava, J. (2010). Chamomile: An herbal medicine of the past with a bright future (Review). Molecular Medicine Reports, 3(6). https://doi.org/10.3892/mmr.2010.377

8. Morssinkhof, M. W. L., van Wylick, D. W., Priester-Vink, S., van der Werf, Y. D., den Heijer, M., van den Heuvel, O. A., & Broekman, B. F. P. (2020). Associations between sex hormones, sleep problems and depression: A systematic review. Neuroscience and biobehavioral reviews, 118, 669–680.

9. Papadopol V, Nechifor M. Magnesium in neuroses and neuroticism. In: Vink R, Nechifor M, editors. Magnesium in the Central Nervous System [Internet]. Adelaide (AU): University of Adelaide Press; 2011. Available from: https://www.ncbi.nlm.nih.gov/books/NBK507254/

10. Qiu, Y., Mao, Z. J., Ruan, Y. P., & Zhang, X. (2021). Exploration of the anti-insomnia mechanism of Ganoderma by central-peripheral multi-level interaction network analysis. BMC microbiology, 21(1), 296. https://doi.org/10.1186/s12866-021-02361-5

11. Rusch, H. L., Rosario, M., Levison, L. M., Olivera, A., Livingston, W. S., Wu, T., & Gill, J. M. (2019). The effect of mindfulness meditation on sleep quality: a systematic review and meta-analysis of randomized controlled trials. Annals of the New York Academy of Sciences, 1445(1), 5–16. https://doi.org/10.1111/nyas.13996

12. Yao, C., Wang, Z., Jiang, H., Yan, R., Huang, Q., & Wang, Y. et al. (2021). Ganoderma lucidum promotes sleep through a gut microbiota-dependent and serotonin-involved pathway in mice. Scientific Reports, 11(1). https://doi.org/10.1038/s41598-021-92913-6

13. Zhang, X., Yin, J., Sun, X., Qu, Z., Zhang, J., & Zhang, H. (2024). The association between insomnia and cognitive decline: A scoping review. Sleep Medicine, 124, 540–550. https://doi.org/10.1016/j.sleep.2024.10.021
14. Zhang, Y., Chen, C., Lu, L., Knutson, K. L., Carnethon, M. R., Fly, A. D., Luo, J., Haas, D. M., Shikany, J. M., & Kahe, K. (2022). Association of magnesium intake with sleep duration and sleep quality: findings from the CARDIA study. Sleep, 45(4), zsab276. https://doi.org/10.1093/sleep/zsab276
15. Zisapel N. (2018). New perspectives on the role of melatonin in human sleep, circadian rhythms and their regulation. British journal of pharmacology, 175(16), 3190–3199. https://doi.org/10.1111/bph.14116

The Mental and Emotional Load of Motherhood

1. Barba-Müller, E., Craddock, S., Carmona, S., & Hoekzema, E. (2019). Brain plasticity in pregnancy and the postpartum period: links to maternal care-giving and mental health. Archives of women's mental health, 22(2), 289–299. https://doi.org/10.1007/s00737-018-0889-z
2. Belliveau, R., Horton, S., Hereford, C., Ridpath, L., Foster, R., & Boothe, E. (2022). Pro-inflammatory diet and depressive symptoms in the healthcare setting. BMC Psychiatry, 22(1). https://doi.org/10.1186/s12888-022-03771-z
3. Busby, E., Bold, J., Fellows, L., & Rostami, K. (2018). Mood Disorders and Gluten: It's Not All in Your Mind! A Systematic Review with Meta-Analysis. Nutrients, 10(11), 1708. https://doi.org/10.3390/nu10111708
4. CDC. (2023, October 13). Mental health conditions: Depression and anxiety. Centers for Disease Control and Prevention; Centers for Disease Control and Prevention. https://www.cdc.gov/tobacco/campaign/tips/diseases/depression-anxiety.html
5. Chang, C. Y., Ke, D. S., & Chen, J. Y. (2009). Essential fatty acids and human brain. Acta Neurologica Taiwanica, 18(4), 231-241.
6. Chao, L., Liu, C., Sutthawongwadee, S., Li, Y., Lv, W., Chen, W., Yu,

L., Zhou, J., Guo, A., Li, Z., & Guo, S. (2020). Effects of Probiotics on Depressive or Anxiety Variables in Healthy Participants Under Stress Conditions or With a Depressive or Anxiety Diagnosis: A Meta-Analysis of Randomized Controlled Trials. Frontiers in neurology, 11, 421. https://doi.org/10.3389/fneur.2020.00421

7. Jacka, F.N., O'Neil, A., Opie, R. et al. A randomized controlled trial of dietary improvement for adults with major depression (the 'SMILES' trial). BMC Med 15, 23 (2017). https://doi.org/10.1186/s12916-017-0791-y

8. Lin, K., Li, Y., Toit, E. D., Wendt, L., & Sun, J. (2021). Effects of Polyphenol Supplementations on Improving Depression, Anxiety, and Quality of Life in Patients with Depression. Frontiers in Psychiatry, 12. https://doi.org/10.3389/fpsyt.2021.765485

9. Ma, T., Jin, H., Kwok, L.-Y., Sun, Z., Liong, M.-T., & Zhang, H. (2021). Probiotic consumption relieved human stress and anxiety symptoms possibly via modulating the neuroactive potential of the gut microbiota. Neurobiology of Stress, 14, 100294. https://doi.org/10.1016/j.ynstr.2021.100294

10. Mandolesi, L., Polverino, A., Montuori, S., Foti, F., Ferraioli, G., Sorrentino, P., & Sorrentino, G. (2018). Effects of Physical Exercise on Cognitive Functioning and Wellbeing: Biological and Psychological Benefits. Frontiers in psychology, 9, 509. https://doi.org/10.3389/fpsyg.2018.00509

11. McLoughlin, E., Arnold, R., & Moore, L. J. (2023). The tendency to appraise stressful situations as more of a threat is associated with poorer health and well-being. Stress and Health, 40(3). https://doi.org/10.1002/smi.3358

12. Modak, A., Ronghe, V., Gomase, K. P., Mahakalkar, M. G., & Taksande, V. (2023). A Comprehensive Review of Motherhood and Mental Health: Postpartum Mood Disorders in Focus. Cureus, 15(9), e46209. https://doi.org/10.7759/cureus.46209

13. Molina-Infante, J., Santolaria, S., Sanders, D. S., & Fernández-Bañares, F. (2015). Systematic review: noncoeliac gluten sensitivity. Alimentary

pharmacology & therapeutics, 41(9), 807–820. https://doi.org/10.1111/apt.13155
14. Reich-Stiebert, N., Froehlich, L., & Voltmer, J. B. (2023). Gendered Mental Labor: A Systematic Literature Review on the Cognitive Dimension of Unpaid Work Within the Household and Childcare. Sex roles, 88(11-12), 475–494. https://doi.org/10.1007/s11199-023-01362-0
15. Reveley, S. (2019). Becoming Mum: Exploring the Emergence and Formulation of a Mother's Identity During the Transition into Motherhood. Childbearing and the Changing Nature of Parenthood: The Contexts, Actors, and Experiences of Having Children, 14, 23–51. https://doi.org/10.1108/s1530-353520190000014002
16. Samtleben, C., & Müller, K.-U. (2021). Care and careers: Gender (in)equality in Unpaid care, Housework and Employment. Research in Social Stratification and Mobility, 77, 100659. https://doi.org/10.1016/j.rssm.2021.100659 Nowland, R., Thomson, G., Cross, L., Whittaker, K., Gregory, P., Charles, J. M., & Day, C. (2023). Exploring blog narratives of parental loneliness: A thematic network analysis. Current Research in Behavioral Sciences, 100137. https://doi.org/10.1016/j.crbeha.2023.100137
17. World Health Organization (2021). Depression. [online] World Health Organization. Available at: https://www.who.int/news-room/fact-sheets/detail/depression.
18. World Health Organization. (2022). WHO guide for integration of perinatal mental health in maternal and child health services. Www.who.int. https://www.who.int/publications/i/item/9789240057142

Navigating Anxiety in Motherhood

1. El Dib, R., Periyasamy, A. G., de Barros, J. L., França, C. G., Senefonte, F. L., Vesentini, G., Alves, M. G. O., Rodrigues, J. V. D. S., Gomaa, H., Gomes Júnior, J. R., Costa, L. F., Von Ancken, T. S., Toneli, C., Suzumura, E. A., Kawakami, C. P., Faustino, E. G., Jorge, E. C., Almeida, J. D., & Kapoor, A. (2021). Probiotics for the treatment of depression and anxiety: A

systematic review and meta-analysis of randomized controlled trials. Clinical nutrition ESPEN, 45, 75–90. https://doi.org/10.1016/j.clnesp.2021.07.027

2. American Psychological Association. (n.d.). Exercise and stress: Get moving to manage stress. Retrieved from https://www.apa.org/topics/exercise-fitness/stress

3. Firth, J., Gangwisch, J. E., Borsini, A., Wootton, R. E., & Mayer, E. A. (2020). Food and mood: How do diet and nutrition affect mental well-being? BMJ, 369, m2382. https://doi.org/10.1136/bmj.m2382

4. Foster, J. A., & McVey Neufeld, K.-A. (2013). Gut–brain axis: How the microbiome influences anxiety and depression. Trends in Neurosciences, 36(5), 305–312. https://doi.org/10.1016/j.tins.2013.01.005

5. Gallup, Inc. (2022). State of the Global Workplace: 2022 Report. Retrieved from https://www.gallup.com

6. Jacka, F. N., O'Neil, A., Opie, R., Itsiopoulos, C., Cotton, S., Mohebbi, M., ... & Berk, M. (2017). A randomized controlled trial of dietary improvement for adults with major depression (the "SMILES" trial). BMC Medicine, 15(1), 23. https://doi.org/10.1186/s12916-017-0791-y

7. Shohani, M., Badfar, G., Nasirkandy, M. P., Kaikhavani, S., Rahmati, S., Modmeli, Y., Soleymani, A., & Azami, M. (2018). The Effect of Yoga on Stress, Anxiety, and Depression in Women. International journal of preventive medicine, 9, 21. https://doi.org/10.4103/ijpvm.IJPVM_242_16

8. Lebel, C., MacKinnon, A., Bagshawe, M., Tomfohr-Madsen, L., & Giesbrecht, G. (2020). Elevated depression and anxiety symptoms among pregnant individuals during the COVID-19 pandemic. Journal of Affective Disorders, 277, 5–13. https://doi.org/10.1016/j.jad.2020.07.126

9. Marotta, A., Sarno, E., Del Casale, A., Pane, M., Mogna, L., Amoruso, A., Felis, G. E., & Fiorio, M. (2019). Effects of Probiotics on Cognitive Reactivity, Mood, and Sleep Quality. Frontiers in psychiatry, 10, 164. https://doi.org/10.3389/fpsyt.2019.00164

10. National Institute of Mental Health. (2022). Anxiety disorders. National

Institutes of Health. Retrieved from https://www.nimh.nih.gov
11. Tamayo, M., Agusti, A., Molina-Mendoza, G. V., Rossini, V., Frances-Cuesta, C., Tolosa-Enguís, V., & Sanz, Y. (2025). Bifidobacterium longum CECT 30763 improves depressive- and anxiety-like behavior in a social defeat mouse model through the immune and dopaminergic systems. Brain, Behavior, and Immunity, 125, 35–57. https://doi.org/10.1016/j.bbi.2024.12.028
12. McCabe, D., Lisy, K., Lockwood, C., & Colbeck, M. (2017). The impact of essential fatty acid, B vitamins, vitamin C, magnesium and zinc supplementation on stress levels in women: a systematic review. JBI database of systematic reviews and implementation reports, 15(2), 402–453. https://doi.org/10.11124/JBISRIR-2016-002965
13. Bistas, K. G., & Tabet, J. P. (2023). The Benefits of Prebiotics and Probiotics on Mental Health. Cureus, 15(8), e43217. https://doi.org/10.7759/cureus.43217
14. Strandwitz, P. (2018). Neurotransmitter modulation by the gut microbiota. Brain Research, 1693, 128–133. https://doi.org/10.1016/j.brainres.2018.03.015
15. Merkouris, E., Mavroudi, T., Miliotas, D., Tsiptsios, D., Serdari, A., Christidi, F., Doskas, T. K., Mueller, C., & Tsamakis, K. (2024). Probiotics' Effects in the Treatment of Anxiety and Depression: A Comprehensive Review of 2014-2023 Clinical Trials. Microorganisms, 12(2), 411. https://doi.org/10.3390/microorganisms12020411
16. Watanabe, T., Abe, S., & Shimada, H. (2021). The effects of structured routines and mindfulness on mental health in parents. Journal of Child Psychology and Psychiatry, 62(3), 314–321. https://doi.org/10.1111/jcpp.13345
17. Kris-Etherton, P. M., Petersen, K. S., Hibbeln, J. R., Hurley, D., Kolick, V., Peoples, S., Rodriguez, N., & Woodward-Lopez, G. (2021). Nutrition and behavioral health disorders: depression and anxiety. Nutrition reviews, 79(3), 247–260. https://doi.org/10.1093/nutrit/nuaa025
18. Woody, C. A., Ferrari, A. J., Siskind, D. J., Whiteford, H. A., & Harris, M. G. (2017). A systematic review and meta-regression of the prevalence and

incidence of perinatal depression. Journal of Affective Disorders, 219, 86–92. https://doi.org/10.1016/j.jad.2017.05.003

19. Bistas, K. G., & Tabet, J. P. (2023). The Benefits of Prebiotics and Probiotics on Mental Health. Cureus, 15(8), e43217. https://doi.org/10.7759/cureus.43217

20. Bertani, D. E., De Novellis, A. M. P., Farina, R., Latella, E., Meloni, M., Scala, C., Valeo, L., Galeazzi, G. M., & Ferrari, S. (2021). "Shedding Light on Light": A Review on the Effects on Mental Health of Exposure to Optical Radiation. International journal of environmental research and public health, 18(4), 1670. https://doi.org/10.3390/ijerph18041670

21. Basiri, R., Seidu, B., & Cheskin, L. J. (2023). Key Nutrients for Optimal Blood Glucose Control and Mental Health in Individuals with Diabetes: A Review of the Evidence. Nutrients, 15(18), 3929. https://doi.org/10.3390/nu15183929

22. Clapp, M., Aurora, N., Herrera, L., Bhatia, M., Wilen, E., & Wakefield, S. (2017). Gut microbiota's effect on mental health: The gut-brain axis. Clinics and practice, 7(4), 987. https://doi.org/10.4081/cp.2017.987

23. MacKay, M., Yang, B. H., Dursun, S. M., & Baker, G. B. (2024). The Gut-Brain Axis and the Microbiome in Anxiety Disorders, Post-Traumatic Stress Disorder and Obsessive-Compulsive Disorder. Current neuropharmacology, 22(5), 866–883. https://doi.org/10.2174/1570159X21666230222092029

24. Balban, M. Y., Neri, E., Kogon, M. M., Weed, L., Nouriani, B., Jo, B., Holl, G., Zeitzer, J. M., Spiegel, D., & Huberman, A. D. (2023). Brief structured respiration practices enhance mood and reduce physiological arousal. Cell reports. Medicine, 4(1), 100895. https://doi.org/10.1016/j.xcrm.2022.100895

25. Lindseth, G., Helland, B., & Caspers, J. (2015). The effects of dietary tryptophan on affective disorders. Archives of psychiatric nursing, 29(2), 102–107. https://doi.org/10.1016/j.apnu.2014.11.008

26. American Psychological Association. (2022, November). Defeating depression naturally: The link between exercise and mental health. APA Monitor. Retrieved from https://www.apa.org/monitor/2022/11/

defeating-depression-naturally

Building a Robust Immune System

1. Abrahams, M., O'Grady, R., & Prawitt, J. (2022). Effect of a Daily Collagen Peptide Supplement on Digestive Symptoms in Healthy Women: 2-Phase Mixed Methods Study. JMIR formative research, 6(5), e36339. https://doi.org/10.2196/36339
2. Charneca, S., Hernando, A., Costa-Reis, P., & Guerreiro, C. S. (2023). Beyond Seasoning-The Role of Herbs and Spices in Rheumatic Diseases. Nutrients, 15(12), 2812. https://doi.org/10.3390/nu15122812
3. Chen, Q., Chen, O., Martins, I. M., Hou, H., Zhao, X., Blumberg, J. B., & Li, B. (2017). Collagen peptides ameliorate intestinal epithelial barrier dysfunction in immunostimulatory Caco-2 cell monolayers via enhancing tight junctions. Food & function, 8(3), 1144–1151. https://doi.org/10.1039/c6fo01347c
4. Daly, J. M., Reynolds, J., Sigal, R. K., Shou, J., & Liberman, M. D. (1990). Effect of dietary protein and amino acids on immune function. Critical care medicine, 18(2 Suppl), S86–S93.
5. Kalogerakou, T., & Antoniadou, M. (2024). The Role of Dietary Antioxidants, Food Supplements and Functional Foods for Energy Enhancement in Healthcare Professionals. Antioxidants, 13(12), 1508. https://doi.org/10.3390/antiox13121508
6. Martínez-Puig, D., Costa-Larrión, E., Rubio-Rodríguez, N., & Gálvez-Martín, P. (2023). Collagen Supplementation for Joint Health: The Link between Composition and Scientific Knowledge. Nutrients, 15(6), 1332. https://doi.org/10.3390/nu15061332
7. National Institutes of Health. (2023, June 27). Office of Dietary Supplements - Dietary Supplements for Immune Function and Infectious Diseases. Ods.od.nih.gov. https://ods.od.nih.gov/factsheets/ImmuneFunction-HealthProfessional/
8. Peters, A., Krumbholz, P., Jäger, E., Heintz-Buschart, A., Çakir, M. V., Rothemund, S., Gaudl, A., Ceglarek, U., Schöneberg, T., & Stäubert, C.

(2019). Metabolites of lactic acid bacteria present in fermented foods are highly potent agonists of human hydroxycarboxylic acid receptor 3. PLOS Genetics, 15(5), e1008145. https://doi.org/10.1371/journal.pgen.1008145

9. Shahbazi, R., Sharifzad, F., Bagheri, R., Alsadi, N., Yasavoli-Sharahi, H., & Matar, C. (2021). Anti-Inflammatory and Immunomodulatory Properties of Fermented Plant Foods. Nutrients, 13(5), 1516. https://doi.org/10.3390/nu13051516
10. Tennant, S. M., Hartland, E. L., Phumoonna, T., Lyras, D., Rood, J. I., Robins-Browne, R. M., & van Driel, I. R. (2008). Influence of gastric acid on susceptibility to infection with ingested bacterial pathogens. Infection and immunity, 76(2), 639–645. https://doi.org/10.1128/IAI.01138-07
11. Tourkochristou, E., Triantos, C., & Mouzaki, A. (2021). The Influence of Nutritional Factors on Immunological Outcomes. Frontiers in Immunology, 12, 665968. https://doi.org/10.3389/fimmu.2021.665968
12. Yagnik, D., Serafin, V., & J Shah, A. (2018). Antimicrobial activity of apple cider vinegar against Escherichia coli, Staphylococcus aureus and Candida albicans; downregulating cytokine and microbial protein expression. Scientific reports, 8(1), 1732. https://doi.org/10.1038/s41598-017-18618-x

Enhance Your Energy

1. Cook J. D. (2005). Diagnosis and management of iron-deficiency anemia. Best practice & research. Clinical haematology, 18(2), 319–332. https://doi.org/10.1016/j.beha.2004.08.022
2. Gröber, U., Schmidt, J., & Kisters, K. (2015). Magnesium in prevention and therapy. Nutrients, 7(9), 8199–8226. https://doi.org/10.3390/nu7095388
3. Hernández-Camacho, J. D., Bernier, M., López-Lluch, G., & Navas, P. (2018). Coenzyme Q10 supplementation in aging and disease. Frontiers

in Physiology, 9, 44. https://doi.org/10.3389/fphys.2018.00044
4. Kreider, R. B., Kalman, D. S., Antonio, J., Ziegenfuss, T. N., Wildman, R., Collins, R., ... & Willoughby, D. S. (2017). International society of sports nutrition position stand: Safety and efficacy of creatine supplementation in exercise, sport, and medicine. Journal of the International Society of Sports Nutrition, 14(1), 18. https://doi.org/10.1186/s12970-017-0173-z
5. Lopresti, A. L., Smith, S. J., Malvi, H., & Kodgule, R. (2019). An investigation into the stress-relieving and pharmacological actions of an ashwagandha (Withania somnifera) extract: A randomized, double-blind, placebo-controlled study. Medicine, 98(37), e17186. https://doi.org/10.1097/MD.0000000000017186
6. O'Leary, F., & Samman, S. (2010). Vitamin B12 in health and disease. Nutrients, 2(3), 299–316. https://doi.org/10.3390/nu2030299
7. Panossian, A., & Wikman, G. (2010). Effects of adaptogens on the central nervous system and the molecular mechanisms associated with their stress-protective activity. Pharmaceuticals, 3(1), 188–224. https://doi.org/10.3390/ph3010188
8. Reay, J. L., Kennedy, D. O., & Scholey, A. B. (2005). Single doses of Panax ginseng (G115) reduce blood glucose levels and improve cognitive performance during sustained mental activity. Journal of Psychopharmacology, 19(4), 357–365. https://doi.org/10.1177/0269881105053286

What's on Your Plate? Why Organic Matters

1. Ahmad, M. F., Fakhruddin Ali Ahmad, Alsayegh, A. A., Md Zeyaullah, AlShahrani, A. M., Khursheed Muzammil, Abdullah Ali Saati, Wahab, S., Elbendary, E. Y., Nahla Kambal, Abdelrahman, M. H., & Hussain, S. (2024). Pesticides impacts on human health and the environment with their mechanisms of action and possible countermeasures. Heliyon, 10(7), e29128–e29128. https://doi.org/10.1016/j.heliyon.2024.e29128
2. Alexanderson, M. S., Luke, H., & Lloyd, D. J. (2024). Regenerative

agriculture in Australia: the changing face of farming. Frontiers in Sustainable Food Systems, 8. https://doi.org/10.3389/fsufs.2024.1402849

3. Ali, A., & AlHussaini, K. I. (2024). Pesticides: Unintended Impact on the Hidden World of Gut Microbiota. Metabolites, 14(3), 155. https://doi.org/10.3390/metabo14030155

4. Barański, M., Srednicka-Tober, D., Volakakis, N., Seal, C., Sanderson, R., Stewart, G. B., Benbrook, C., Biavati, B., Markellou, E., Giotis, C., Gromadzka-Ostrowska, J., Rembiałkowska, E., Skwarło-Sońta, K., Tahvonen, R., Janovská, D., Niggli, U., Nicot, P., & Leifert, C. (2014). Higher antioxidant and lower cadmium concentrations and lower incidence of pesticide residues in organically grown crops: a systematic literature review and meta-analyses. The British journal of nutrition, 112(5), 794–811. https://doi.org/10.1017/S0007114514001366

5. Barański, M., Srednicka-Tober, D., Volakakis, N., Seal, C., Sanderson, R., Stewart, G. B., ... & Leifert, C. (2014). Higher antioxidant and lower cadmium concentrations and lower incidence of pesticide residues in organically grown crops: A systematic literature review and meta-analyses. British Journal of Nutrition, 112(5), 794–811. https://doi.org/10.1017/S0007114514001366

6. Diamanti-Kandarakis, E., Bourguignon, J. P., Giudice, L. C., Hauser, R., Prins, G. S., Soto, A. M., ... & Gore, A. C. (2009). Endocrine-disrupting chemicals: An endocrine society scientific statement. Endocrine Reviews, 30(4), 293-342. https://doi.org/10.1210/er.2009-0002

7. Grand View Research. (2023). Organic food & beverage market size, share & trends analysis report by product, by region, and segment forecasts, 2023 - 2030. Retrieved from https://www.grandviewresearch.com/industry-analysis/organic-foods-beverages-market

8. Kell, D. B. (2012). Large-scale sequestration of atmospheric carbon via plant roots in natural and agricultural ecosystems: Why and how. Philosophical Transactions of the Royal Society B: Biological Sciences, 367(1595), 1589–1597. https://doi.org/10.1098/rstb.2011.0244

9. Khangura, R., Ferris, D., Wagg, C., & Bowyer, J. (2023). Regenerative

Agriculture—A Literature Review on the Practices and Mechanisms Used to Improve Soil Health. Sustainability, 15(3), 2338. https://doi.org/10.3390/su15032338

10. Mnif, W., Hassine, A. I., Bouaziz, A., Bartegi, A., Thomas, O., & Roig, B. (2011). Effect of endocrine disruptor pesticides: a review. International journal of environmental research and public health, 8(6), 2265–2303. https://doi.org/10.3390/ijerph8062265

11. Ramkumar, D., Marty, A., Ramkumar, J., Rosencranz, H., Vedantham, R., Goldman, M., Meyer, E., Steinmetz, J., Weckle, A., Bloedorn, K., & Rosier, C. (2024). Food for thought: Making the case for food produced via regenerative agriculture in the battle against non-communicable chronic diseases (NCDs). One health (Amsterdam, Netherlands), 18, 100734. https://doi.org/10.1016/j.onehlt.2024.100734

12. Rao, T. S., Asha, M. R., Ramesh, B. N., & Rao, K. S. (2008). Understanding nutrition, depression and mental illnesses. Indian journal of psychiatry, 50(2), 77–82. https://doi.org/10.4103/0019-5545.42391

13. Reganold, J. P., & Wachter, J. M. (2016). Organic agriculture in the twenty-first century. Nature Plants, 2(2), 15221. https://doi.org/10.1038/nplants.2015.221

14. Rekha, Naik, S. N., & Prasad, R. (2006). Pesticide residue in organic and conventional food-risk analysis. Journal of Chemical Health and Safety, 13(6), 12–19. https://doi.org/10.1016/j.chs.2005.01.012

15. Sathyanarayana Rao, T., Asha, M., Ramesh, B., & Jagannatha Rao, K. (2008). Understanding nutrition, depression and mental illnesses. Indian Journal of Psychiatry, 50(2), 77. https://doi.org/10.4103/0019-5545.42391

16. Vandenberg, L. N., Colborn, T., Hayes, T. B., Heindel, J. J., Jacobs, D. R., Lee, D. H., & Shioda, T. (2012). Hormones and endocrine-disrupting chemicals: Low-dose effects and nonmonotonic dose responses. Endocrine Reviews, 33(3), 378-455. https://doi.org/10.1210/er.2011-1050

Organic on a Budget: Strategies for Healthier, Low-Pesticide Food Choices

1. Barański, M., Srednicka-Tober, D., Volakakis, N., Seal, C., Sanderson, R., Stewart, G. B., ... & Leifert, C. (2014). Higher antioxidant and lower cadmium concentrations and lower incidence of pesticide residues in organically grown crops: A systematic literature review and meta-analyses. British Journal of Nutrition, 112(5), 794–811. https://doi.org/10.1017/S0007114514001366
2. Birtalan, I. L., Bartha, A., Neulinger, Á., Bárdos, G., Oláh, A., Rácz, J., & Rigó, A. (2020). Community Supported Agriculture as a Driver of Food-Related Well-Being. Sustainability, 12(11), 4516. https://doi.org/10.3390/su12114516
3. Cimmino, I., Fiory, F., Perruolo, G., Miele, C., Beguinot, F., Formisano, P., & Oriente, F. (2020). Potential Mechanisms of Bisphenol A (BPA) Contributing to Human Disease. International journal of molecular sciences, 21(16), 5761. https://doi.org/10.3390/ijms21165761
4. Eng, S., Khun, T., Jower, S., & Murro, M. J. (2019). Healthy Lifestyle Through Home Gardening: The Art of Sharing. American journal of lifestyle medicine, 13(4), 347–350. https://doi.org/10.1177/1559827619842068
5. Environmental Working Group. (2024). EWG's 2021 Shopper's Guide to Pesticides in ProduceTM. EWG. https://www.ewg.org/foodnews/full-list.php
6. Hughner, R. S., McDonagh, P., Prothero, A., Shultz, C. J., & Stanton, J. (2007). Who are organic food consumers? A compilation and review of why people purchase organic food. Journal of Consumer Behaviour, 6(2-3), 94-110. https://doi.org/10.1002/cb.210
7. Kieffer, D. A., Martin, R. J., & Adams, S. H. (2016). Impact of Dietary Fibers on Nutrient Management and Detoxification Organs: Gut, Liver, and Kidneys. Advances in nutrition (Bethesda, Md.), 7(6), 1111–1121. https://doi.org/10.3945/an.116.013219
8. La Merrill, M.A., Vandenberg, L.N., Smith, M.T. et al. Consensus on the key characteristics of endocrine-disrupting chemicals as a basis for hazard identification. Nat Rev Endocrinol 16, 45–57 (2020). https://doi.org/10.1038/s41574-019-0273-8

9. M, M., & Vellapandian, C. (2024). Exploring the Long-Term Effect of Artificial Sweeteners on Metabolic Health. Cureus, 16(9), e70043. https://doi.org/10.7759/cureus.70043
10. Paramasivam, A., Murugan, R., Jeraud, M., Dakkumadugula, A., Periyasamy, R., & Arjunan, S. (2024). Additives in Processed Foods as a Potential Source of Endocrine-Disrupting Chemicals: A Review. Journal of xenobiotics, 14(4), 1697–1710. https://doi.org/10.3390/jox14040090
11. Rickman, J. C., Barrett, D. M., & Bruhn, C. M. (2007). Nutritional comparison of fresh, frozen and canned fruits and vegetables. Part 1. Journal of the Science of Food and Agriculture, 87(6), 930–944. https://doi.org/10.1002/jsfa.2824
12. Seneff, S., & Samsel, A. (2015). Glyphosate, pathways to modern diseases III: Manganese, neurological diseases, and associated pathologies. Surgical Neurology International, 6(1), https://doi.org/10.4103/2152-7806.153876
13. Smith-Spangler, C., Brandeau, M. L., Hunter, G. E., Bavinger, J. C., Pearson, M., Eschbach, P. J., ... & Bravata, D. M. (2012). Are organic foods safer or healthier than conventional alternatives? A systematic review. Annals of Internal Medicine, 157(5), 348-366. https://doi.org/10.7326/0003-4819-157-5-201209040-00007
14. Średnicka-Tober, D., Barański, M., Seal, C. J., Sanderson, R., Benbrook, C., Steinshamn, H., ... & Leifert, C. (2016). Composition differences between organic and conventional meat: A systematic literature review and meta-analysis. British Journal of Nutrition, 115(6), 994–1011. https://doi.org/10.1017/S0007114515005073
15. Zhou, W., Li, M., & Achal, V. (2024). A Comprehensive Review on Environmental and Human Health Impacts of Chemical Pesticide Usage. Emerging Contaminants, 11(1), 100410–100410. https://doi.org/10.1016/j.emcon.2024.100410

Avoiding Harmful Chemicals

1. Balwierz, R., Biernat, P., Jasińska-Balwierz, A., Siodłak, D., Kusakiewicz-Dawid, A., Kurek-Górecka, A., Olczyk, P., & Ochędzan-Siodłak, W. (2023). Potential Carcinogens in Makeup Cosmetics. International journal of environmental research and public health, 20(6), 4780. https://doi.org/10.3390/ijerph20064780
2. Blake, B. E., & Fenton, S. E. (2020). Early life exposure to per- and polyfluoroalkyl substances (PFAS) and latent health outcomes: A review including the placenta as a target tissue and possible driver of peri- and postnatal effects. Toxicology, 443, 152565. https://doi.org/10.1016/j.tox.2020.152565
3. Bocarsly, M. E., Powell, E. S., Avena, N. M., & Hoebel, B. G. (2017). High-fructose corn syrup causes characteristics of obesity in rats: Increased body weight, body fat and triglyceride levels. Pharmacology Biochemistry and Behavior, 97(1), 101-106.
4. Chiu, K., Warner, G., Nowak, R. A., Flaws, J. A., & Mei, W. (2020). The Impact of Environmental Chemicals on the Gut Microbiome. Toxicological sciences: an official journal of the Society of Toxicology, 176(2), 253–284. https://doi.org/10.1093/toxsci/kfaa065
5. Chouhan, S., Sharma, K., & Guleria, S. (2017). Antimicrobial Activity of Some Essential Oils-Present Status and Future Perspectives. Medicines (Basel, Switzerland), 4(3), 58. https://doi.org/10.3390/medicines4030058
6. Crinnion, W. J. (2010). Organic foods contain higher levels of certain nutrients, lower levels of pesticides, and may provide health benefits for the consumer. Alternative Medicine Review, 15(1), 4-12.
7. Darbre, P. D., & Charles, A. K. (2010). Environmental oestrogens and breast cancer: evidence for combined involvement of dietary, household and cosmetic xenoestrogens. Anticancer research, 30(3), 815–827.
8. Environmental Working Group. (2019). Dirty DozenTM Fruits and Vegetables with the Most Pesticides. Environmental Working Group. https://www.ewg.org/foodnews/dirty-dozen.php
9. FDA. (2022, February 25). Parabens in Cosmetics. Fda.gov. https://www.fda.gov/cosmetics/cosmetic-ingredients/parabens-cosmetics

10. Hlisníková, H., Petrovičová, I., Kolena, B., Šidlovská, M., & Sirotkin, A. (2020). Effects and Mechanisms of Phthalates' Action on Reproductive Processes and Reproductive Health: A Literature Review. International journal of environmental research and public health, 17(18), 6811. https://doi.org/10.3390/ijerph17186811
11. Lodén, M., & Maibach, H. I. (2016). Sulfate-free shampoos and skin health: A focus on sodium lauryl sulfate and sodium laureth sulfate. Journal of Clinical Dermatology, 19(4), 13-24.
12. Miller, M. D., Steinmaus, C., Golub, M. S., Castorina, R., Thilakartne, R., Bradman, A., & Marty, M. A. (2022). Potential impacts of synthetic food dyes on activity and attention in children: a review of the human and animal evidence. Environmental health: a global access science source, 21(1), 45. https://doi.org/10.1186/s12940-022-00849-9
13. Mitra, S., Chakraborty, A. J., Tareq, A. M., Emran, T. B., Nainu, F., Khusro, A., Idris, A. M., Khandaker, M. U., Osman, H., Alhumaydhi, F. A., & Simal-Gandara, J. (2022). Impact of Heavy Metals on the Environment and Human health: Novel Therapeutic Insights to Counter the Toxicity. Journal of King Saud University - Science, 34(3), 101865. https://doi.org/10.1016/j.jksus.2022.101865
14. Moon M. K. (2019). Concern about the Safety of Bisphenol A Substitutes. Diabetes & metabolism journal, 43(1), 46–48. https://doi.org/10.4093/dmj.2019.0027
15. Naidu, R., Biswas, B., Willet, I., Cribb, J., & Singh, B. (2021). Chemical pollution: A growing peril and potential catastrophic risk to humanity. Environment International, 156, 106616. https://doi.org/10.1016/j.envint.2021.106616
16. National Cancer Institute. (2021). Formaldehyde and cancer risk. Retrieved from https://www.cancer.gov/about-cancer/causes-prevention/risk/substances/formaldehyde/formaldehyde-fact-sheet
17. National Institute of Environmental Health Sciences. (2023, March 9). Perfluoroalkyl and Polyfluoroalkyl Substances (PFAS). National Institute of Environmental Health Sciences. https://www.niehs.nih.gov/health/topics/agents/pfc/index.cfm

18. Rádis-Baptista, G. (2023). Do Synthetic Fragrances in Personal Care and Household Products Impact Indoor Air Quality and Pose Health Risks? Journal of Xenobiotics, 13(1), 121–131. https://doi.org/10.3390/jox13010010
19. Sun, C., Zhang, T., Zhou, Y., Liu, Z., Zhang, Y., Bian, Y., & Feng, X. (2023). Triclosan and related compounds in the environment: Recent updates on sources, fates, distribution, analytical extraction, analysis, and removal techniques. Science of the Total Environment, 870, 161885. https://doi.org/10.1016/j.scitotenv.2023.161885
20. Svanes, O., Bertelsen, R. J., Lygre, S. H., & et al. (2018). Cleaning at home and at work in relation to lung function decline and airway obstruction. American Journal of Respiratory and Critical Care Medicine, 197(9), 1157-1163.
21. Toxicological Profile for Ammonia. Atlanta (GA): Agency for Toxic Substances and Disease Registry (US); 2004 Sep. 3, HEALTH EFFECTS. Available from: https://www.ncbi.nlm.nih.gov/books/NBK598714/
22. Wdowiak, N., Wójtowicz, K., Wdowiak-Filip, A., Pucek, W., Wróbel, A., Wróbel, J., & Wdowiak, A. (2024). Environmental Factors as the Main Hormonal Disruptors of Male Fertility. Journal of clinical medicine, 13(7), 1986. https://doi.org/10.3390/jcm13071986

Detoxing for Health: Understanding the Basics

1. Ahmad, R. S., Hussain, M. B., Sultan, M. T., Arshad, M. S., Waheed, M., Shariati, M. A., Plygun, S., & Hashempur, M. H. (2020). Biochemistry, Safety, Pharmacological Activities, and Clinical Applications of Turmeric: A Mechanistic Review. Evidence-based complementary and alternative medicine: eCAM, 2020, 7656919. https://doi.org/10.1155/2020/7656919
2. Ahn, J. Y., Kim, J., Cheong, D. H., Hong, H., Jeong, J. Y., & Kim, B. G. (2022). An In Vitro Study on the Efficacy of Mycotoxin Sequestering Agents for Aflatoxin B1, Deoxynivalenol, and Zearalenone. Animals: an open access journal from MDPI, 12(3), 333. https://doi.org/10.3390/

ani12030333

3. Beretta, G., & Shala, A. L. (2022). Impact of Heat Shock Proteins in Neurodegeneration: Possible Therapeutical Targets. Annals of Neurosciences, 0972753121110705. https://doi.org/10.1177/09727531211070528

4. Bevilacqua, A., Campaniello, D., Speranza, B., Racioppo, A., Sinigaglia, M., & Corbo, M. R. (2024). An Update on Prebiotics and on Their Health Effects. Foods (Basel, Switzerland), 13(3), 446. https://doi.org/10.3390/foods13030446

5. Bibbins-Domingo, K., Grossman, D. C., Curry, S. J., Davidson, K. W., Epling, J. W., García, F. A., ... & Pignone, M. P. (2016). Screening for colorectal cancer: US Preventive Services Task Force recommendation statement. JAMA, 315(23), 2564-2575. https://doi.org/10.1001/jama.2016.5989

6. Bito, T., Okumura, E., Fujishima, M., & Watanabe, F. (2020). Potential of Chlorella as a Dietary Supplement to Promote Human Health. Nutrients, 12(9), 2524. https://doi.org/10.3390/nu12092524

7. Bosetti, C., Filomeno, M., Riso, P., Polesel, J., Levi, F., Talamini, R., Montella, M., Negri, E., Franceschi, S., & La Vecchia, C. (2012). Cruciferous vegetables and cancer risk in a network of case-control studies. Annals of oncology: official journal of the European Society for Medical Oncology, 23(8), 2198–2203.

8. Carr, A. C., & Frei, B. (1999). Toward a new recommended dietary allowance for vitamin C based on antioxidant and health effects in humans. The American journal of clinical nutrition, 69(6), 1086–1107. https://doi.org/10.1093/ajcn/69.6.1086

9. Centers for Disease Control and Prevention (CDC), National Center for Environmental Health. (n.d.). *National biomonitoring program*. Retrieved June 16, 2025, from https://www.cdc.gov/biomonitoring

10. Chacko, S. M., Thambi, P. T., Kuttan, R., & Nishigaki, I. (2010). Beneficial effects of green tea: a literature review. Chinese medicine, 5, 13. https://doi.org/10.1186/1749-8546-5-13

11. Chandrasekaran, P., Weiskirchen, S., & Weiskirchen, R. (2024). Effects

of Probiotics on Gut Microbiota: An Overview. International journal of molecular sciences, 25(11), 6022. https://doi.org/10.3390/ijms25116022

12. Chen, L., Zhu, Y., Hu, Z., Wu, S., & Jin, C. (2021). Beetroot as a functional food with huge health benefits: Antioxidant, antitumor, physical function, and chronic metabolomics activity. Food science & nutrition, 9(11), 6406–6420. https://doi.org/10.1002/fsn3.2577

13. Cueni, L. N., & Detmar, M. (2008). The lymphatic system in health and disease. Lymphatic research and biology, 6(3-4), 109–122. https://doi.org/10.1089/lrb.2008.1008

14. Elmaghraby, D. A., Alsalman, G. A., Alawadh, L. H., Al-Abdulqader, S. A., Alaithan, M. M., & Alnuwaysir, B. I. (2023). Integrated traditional herbal medicine in the treatment of gastrointestinal disorder: the pattern of use and the knowledge of safety among the Eastern Region Saudi population. BMC complementary medicine and therapies, 23(1), 373. https://doi.org/10.1186/s12906-023-04197-0

15. Emadi, S. A., Ghasemzadeh Rahbardar, M., Mehri, S., & Hosseinzadeh, H. (2022). A review of therapeutic potentials of milk thistle (Silybum marianum L.) and its main constituent, silymarin, on cancer, and their related patents. Iranian journal of basic medical sciences, 25(10), 1166–1176. https://doi.org/10.22038/IJBMS.2022.63200.13961

16. Eve, A. A., Liu, X., Wang, Y., Miller, M. J., Jeffery, E. H., & Madak-Erdogan, Z. (2020). Biomarkers of Broccoli Consumption: Implications for Glutathione Metabolism and Liver Health. Nutrients, 12(9), 2514. https://doi.org/10.3390/nu12092514

17. Febbraio F. (2017). Biochemical strategies for the detection and detoxification of toxic chemicals in the environment. World journal of biological chemistry, 8(1), 13–20. https://doi.org/10.4331/wjbc.v8.i1.13

18. Genuis, S. J., Beesoon, S., Birkholz, D., & Lobo, R. A. (2012). Human excretion of bisphenol A: blood, urine, and sweat (BUS) study. Journal of environmental and public health, 2012, 185731. https://doi.org/10.1155/2012/185731

19. Glibowski P. (2020). Organic food and health. Roczniki Panstwowego

Zakladu Higieny, 71(2), 131–136. https://doi.org/10.32394/rpzh.2020.0110

20. Green, C. J., & Hodson, L. (2014). The influence of dietary fat on liver fat accumulation. Nutrients, 6(11), 5018–5033. https://doi.org/10.3390/nu6115018

21. Huang, C. B., Alimova, Y., Myers, T. M., & Ebersole, J. L. (2011). Short- and medium-chain fatty acids exhibit antimicrobial activity for oral microorganisms. Archives of oral biology, 56(7), 650–654. https://doi.org/10.1016/j.archoralbio.2011.01.01

22. Hussain, J., & Cohen, M. (2018). Clinical effects of regular dry sauna bathing: A systematic review. Evidence-Based Complementary and Alternative Medicine, 2018, 1-10. https://doi.org/10.1155/2018/1857413

23. Jalali, M., Mahmoodi, M., Mosallanezhad, Z., Jalali, R., Imanieh, M. H., & Moosavian, S. P. (2020). The effects of curcumin supplementation on liver function, metabolic profile and body composition in patients with non-alcoholic fatty liver disease: A systematic review and meta-analysis of randomized controlled trials. Complementary Therapies in Medicine, 48, 102283. https://doi.org/10.1016/j.ctim.2019.102283

24. Johnson, S. E., & Sherding, R. G. (2006). Diseases of the Liver and Biliary Tract. Saunders Manual of Small Animal Practice, 747–809. https://doi.org/10.1016/B0-72-160422-6/50073-5

25. Kania-Dobrowolska, M., & Baraniak, J. (2022). Dandelion (Taraxacum officinale L.) as a Source of Biologically Active Compounds Supporting the Therapy of Co-Existing Diseases in Metabolic Syndrome. Foods (Basel, Switzerland), 11(18), 2858. https://doi.org/10.3390/foods11182858

26. Khanna, R., MacDonald, J. K., & Levesque, B. G. (2014). Peppermint oil for the treatment of irritable bowel syndrome: a systematic review and meta-analysis. Journal of clinical gastroenterology, 48(6), 505–512. https://doi.org/10.1097/MCG.0b013e3182a88357

27. Kostiuchenko, O., Kravchenko, N., Markus, J., Burleigh, S., Fedkiv, O., Cao, L., Letasiova, S., Skibo, G., Fåk Hållenius, F., & Prykhodko, O. (2022). Effects of Proteases from Pineapple and Papaya on Protein Digestive

Capacity and Gut Microbiota in Healthy C57BL/6 Mice and Dose-Manner Response on Mucosal Permeability in Human Reconstructed Intestinal 3D Tissue Model. Metabolites, 12(11), 1027. https://doi.org/10.3390/metabo12111027

28. Laukkanen, J. A., Laukkanen, T., & Kunutsor, S. K. (2018). Cardiovascular and Other Health Benefits of Sauna Bathing: A Review of the Evidence. Mayo Clinic Proceedings, 93(8), 1111–1121. https://doi.org/10.1016/j.mayocp.2018.04.008

29. Laukkanen, T., Khan, H., Zaccardi, F., & Laukkanen, J. A. (2015). Association between sauna bathing and fatal cardiovascular and all-cause mortality events. JAMA internal medicine, 175(4), 542–548. https://doi.org/10.1001/jamainternmed.2014.8187

30. Lavezzi, A. M., & Ramos-Molina, B. (2023). Environmental Exposure Science and Human Health. International journal of environmental research and public health, 20(10), 5764. https://doi.org/10.3390/ijerph20105764

31. Li, Y., Chen, Y., & Sun-Waterhouse, D. (2022). The potential of dandelion in the fight against gastrointestinal diseases: A review. Journal of Ethnopharmacology, 293, 115272. https://doi.org/10.1016/j.jep.2022.115272

32. Xing, L., Fu, L., Cao, S., Yin, Y., Wei, L., & Zhang, W. (2022). The Anti-Inflammatory Effect of Bovine Bone-Gelatin-Derived Peptides in LPS-Induced RAW264.7 Macrophages Cells and Dextran Sulfate Sodium-Induced C57BL/6 Mice. *Nutrients*, 14(7), 1479. https://doi.org/10.3390/nu14071479

33. Lim, J., Henry, C. J., & Haldar, S. (2016). Vinegar as a functional ingredient to improve postprandial glycemic control-human intervention findings and molecular mechanisms. Molecular nutrition & food research, 60(8), 1837–1849. https://doi.org/10.1002/mnfr.201600121

34. Longo, V. D., & Mattson, M. P. (2014). Fasting: molecular mechanisms and clinical applications. Cell metabolism, 19(2), 181–192. https://doi.org/10.1016/j.cmet.2013.12.008

35. Maiuolo, J., Musolino, V., Gliozzi, M., Carresi, C., Scarano, F., Nucera, S.,

Scicchitano, M., Oppedisano, F., Bosco, F., Macri, R., Palma, E., Muscoli, C., & Mollace, V. (2022). Involvement of the Intestinal Microbiota in the Appearance of Multiple Sclerosis: Aloe vera and Citrus bergamia as Potential Candidates for Intestinal Health. Nutrients, 14(13), 2711. https://doi.org/10.3390/nu14132711

36. Martinez-Lopez, N., Tarabra, E., Toledo, M., Garcia-Macia, M., Sahu, S., Coletto, L., Batista-Gonzalez, A., Barzilai, N., Pessin, J. E., Schwartz, G. J., Kersten, S., & Singh, R. (2017). System-wide Benefits of Intermeal Fasting by Autophagy. Cell metabolism, 26(6), 856–871.e5. https://doi.org/10.1016/j.cmet.2017.09.020

37. Mathers J. C. (2023). Dietary fiber and health: the story so far. The Proceedings of the Nutrition Society, 82(2), 120–129. https://doi.org/10.1017/S0029665123002215

38. Miquel-Kergoat, S., Azais-Braesco, V., Burton-Freeman, B., & Hetherington, M. M. (2015). Effects of chewing on appetite, food intake and gut hormones: A systematic review and meta-analysis. Physiology & behavior, 151, 88–96. https://doi.org/10.1016/j.physbeh.2015.07.017

39. Muir, D. C. G., Getzinger, G. J., McBride, M., & Ferguson, P. L. (2023). How Many Chemicals in Commerce Have Been Analyzed in Environmental Media? A 50 Year Bibliometric Analysis. Environmental science & technology, 57(25), 9119–9129. https://doi.org/10.1021/acs.est.2c09353

40. Mukherji, A., Bailey, S. M., Staels, B., & Baumert, T. F. (2019). The circadian clock and liver function in health and disease. Journal of hepatology, 71(1), 200–211. https://doi.org/10.1016/j.jhep.2019.03.020

41. Nihart, A. J., Garcia, M. A., El Hayek, E., Liu, R., Olewine, M., Kingston, J. D., Castillo, E. F., Gullapalli, R. R., Howard, T., Bleske, B., Scott, J., Gonzalez-Estrella, J., Gross, J. M., Spilde, M., Adolphi, N. L., Gallego, D. F., Jarrell, H. S., Dvorscak, G., Zuluaga-Ruiz, M. E., & West, A. B. (2025). Bioaccumulation of microplastics in decedent human brains. Nature Medicine, 31. https://doi.org/10.1038/s41591-024-03453-1

42. Padula, A. M., Monk, C., Brennan, P. A., Borders, A., Barrett, E. S., McEvoy, C. T., Foss, S., Desai, P., Alshawabkeh, A., Wurth, R., Salafia, C., Fichorova, R., Varshavsky, J., Kress, A., Woodruff, T. J., Morello-

Frosch, R., & program collaborators for Environmental influences on Child Health Outcomes (2020). A review of maternal prenatal exposures to environmental chemicals and psychosocial stressors-implications for research on perinatal outcomes in the ECHO program. Journal of perinatology: official journal of the California Perinatal Association, 40(1), 10–24. https://doi.org/10.1038/s41372-019-0510-y

43. Palmisano, B. T., Zhu, L., & Stafford, J. M. (2017). Role of Estrogens in the Regulation of Liver Lipid Metabolism. Advances in experimental medicine and biology, 1043, 227–256. https://doi.org/10.1007/978-3-319-70178-3_12

44. Patrick, R. P., & Johnson, T. L. (2021). Sauna use as a lifestyle practice to extend healthspan. Experimental Gerontology, 154, 111509. https://doi.org/10.1016/j.exger.2021.111509 Thompson, W. R., Sallis, R., Joy, E., Jaworski, C. A., Stuhr, R. M., & Trilk, J. L. (2020). Exercise Is Medicine. American journal of lifestyle medicine, 14(5), 511–523. https://doi.org/10.1177/1559827620912192

45. Pfingstgraf, I. O., Taulescu, M., Pop, R. M., Orăsan, R., Vlase, L., Uifalean, A., Todea, D., Alexescu, T., Toma, C., & Pârvu, A. E. (2021). Protective Effects of Taraxacum officinale L. (Dandelion) Root Extract in Experimental Acute on Chronic Liver Failure. Antioxidants (Basel, Switzerland), 10(4), 504. https://doi.org/10.3390/antiox10040504

46. Pradhan, S., Blanton, C., Ochoa-Reparaz, J., Bhattarai, N., & Sharma, K. (2024). Herbs and Spices: Modulation of Gut Microbiota for Healthy Aging. Gastroenterology Insights, 15(2), 447–458. https://doi.org/10.3390/gastroent15020032

47. Ragusa, A., Svelato, A., Santacroce, C., Catalano, P., Notarstefano, V., Carnevali, O., Papa, F., Rongioletti, M. C. A., Baiocco, F., Draghi, S., D'Amore, E., Rinaldo, D., Matta, M., & Giorgini, E. (2021). Plasticenta: First evidence of microplastics in human placenta. *Environment International, 146*, 106274. https://doi.org/10.1016/j.envint.2020.106274

48. Rajendran, P., Rengarajan, T., Thangavel, J., Nishigaki, I., Sakthisekaran, D., Sethi, G., & Nishigaki, Y. (2014). The vascular endothelium and human diseases. International Journal of Biological

Sciences, 9(10), 1057-1069. https://doi.org/10.7150/ijbs.7502
49. Rezaie, P., Bitarafan, V., Horowitz, M., & Feinle-Bisset, C. (2021). Effects of Bitter Substances on GI Function, Energy Intake and Glycaemia-Do Preclinical Findings Translate to Outcomes in Humans? Nutrients, 13(4), 1317. https://doi.org/10.3390/nu13041317
50. Schwenger, K. J., Clermont-Dejean, N., & Allard, J. P. (2019). The role of the gut microbiome in chronic liver disease: the clinical evidence revised. JHEP reports: innovation in hepatology, 1(3), 214–226. https://doi.org/10.1016/j.jhepr.2019.04.004
51. Slavin J. (2013). Fiber and prebiotics: mechanisms and health benefits. Nutrients, 5(4), 1417–1435. https://doi.org/10.3390/nu5041417
52. Sutton, P., Woodruff, T. J., Perron, J., Stotland, N., Conry, J. A., Miller, M. D., & Giudice, L. C. (2012). Toxic environmental chemicals: the role of reproductive health professionals in preventing harmful exposures. American journal of obstetrics and gynecology, 207(3), 164–173. https://doi.org/10.1016/j.ajog.2012.01.034
53. Trasande, L. (2019). *Sicker, fatter, poorer : the urgent threat of hormone-disrupting chemicals to our health and future ... and what we can do about it.* Houghton Mifflin Harcourt.
54. Visioli, F., Mucignat-Caretta, C., Anile, F., & Panaite, S. A. (2022). Traditional and Medical Applications of Fasting. Nutrients, 14(3), 433. https://doi.org/10.3390/nu14030433
55. Wang, Z., Walker, G. W., Muir, D. C. G., & Nagatani-Yoshida, K. (2020). Toward a Global Understanding of Chemical Pollution: A First Comprehensive Analysis of National and Regional Chemical Inventories. *Environmental Science & Technology*, 54(5), 2575–2584. https://doi.org/10.1021/acs.est.9b06379
56. Whitsett, M., & VanWagner, L. B. (2015). Physical activity as a treatment of non-alcoholic fatty liver disease: A systematic review. World journal of hepatology, 7(16), 2041–2052. https://doi.org/10.4254/wjh.v7.i16.2041
57. Xu, M.-Y., Guo, C.-C., Li, M.-Y., Lou, Y.-H., Chen, Z.-R., Liu, B.-W., & Lan, L. (2022). Brain-gut-liver axis: Chronic psychological stress

promotes liver injury and fibrosis via gut in rats. Frontiers in Cellular and Infection Microbiology, 12. https://doi.org/10.3389/fcimb.2022.1040749

The Role of Exercise in Postpartum Recovery

1. Chtourou, H., & Souissi, N. (2012). The effect of training at a specific time of day: a review. Journal of strength and conditioning research, 26(7), 1984–2005. https://doi.org/10.1519/JSC.0b013e31825770a7
2. Copeland, J. L., Consitt, L. A., & Tremblay, M. S. (2002). Hormonal Responses to Endurance and Resistance Exercise in Females Aged 19-69 Years. The Journals of Gerontology Series A: Biological Sciences and Medical Sciences, 57(4), B158–B165. https://doi.org/10.1093/gerona/57.4.b158
3. Domingos, C., Pêgo, J. M., & Santos, N. C. (2021). Effects of physical activity on brain function and structure in older adults: A systematic review. Behavioural brain research, 402, 113061. https://doi.org/10.1016/j.bbr.2020.113061
4. Evenson, K. R., Brown, W. J., Brinson, A. K., Budzynski-Seymour, E., & Hayman, M. (2023). A review of public health guidelines for postpartum physical activity and sedentary behavior from around the world. Journal of Sport and Health Science. https://doi.org/10.1016/j.jshs.2023.12.004
5. Koblinsky, N. D., Power, K. A., Middleton, L., Ferland, G., & Anderson, N. D. (2023). The Role of the Gut Microbiome in Diet and Exercise Effects on Cognition: A Review of the Intervention Literature. The journals of gerontology. Series A, Biological sciences and medical sciences, 78(2), 195–205. https://doi.org/10.1093/gerona/glac166
6. Phillips C. (2017). Lifestyle Modulators of Neuroplasticity: How Physical Activity, Mental Engagement, and Diet Promote Cognitive Health during Aging. Neural plasticity, 2017, 3589271. https://doi.org/10.1155/2017/3589271
7. Schoenfeld B. J. (2010). The mechanisms of muscle hypertrophy and their application to resistance training. Journal of strength and

conditioning research, 24(10), 2857–2872. https://doi.org/10.1519/JSC.0b013e3181e840f3

Personalized Nutrition & Health Plans

1. Celis-Morales, C., Livingstone, K. M., Marsaux, C. F. M., Macready, A. L., Fallaize, R., O'Donovan, C. B., ... & Lovegrove, J. A. (2017). Effect of personalized nutrition on health-related behavior change: evidence from the Food4Me European randomized controlled trial. International Journal of Epidemiology, 46(2), 578–588. https://doi.org/10.1093/ije/dyw186
2. Horne, J., Gillies, C., Maher, J., Maddock, J., Stradling, J., & Matthews, P. (2021). Weight management and personalized nutrition: Barriers and facilitators in primary care settings. Nutrition Bulletin, 46(3), 317–325. https://doi.org/10.1111/nbu.12522
3. Konstantinidou, V., Daimiel, L., & Ordovás, J. M. (2014). Personalized nutrition and cardiovascular disease prevention: From Framingham to PREDIMED. Advances in nutrition (Bethesda, Md.), 5(3), 368S–71S. https://doi.org/10.3945/an.113.005686
4. Ordovas, J. M., Ferguson, L. R., Tai, E. S., & Mathers, J. C. (2018). Personalized nutrition and health. BMJ, 361, k2173. https://doi.org/10.1136/bmj.k2173
5. Sarris, J., Logan, A. C., Akbaraly, T. N., Amminger, G. P., Balanz\u00e1-Mart\u00ednez, V., Freeman, M. P., ... & Mischoulon, D. (2015). Nutritional medicine as mainstream in psychiatry. The Lancet Psychiatry, 2(3), 271–274. https://doi.org/10.1016/S2215-0366(14)00051-0
6. Vrolix, R., & Mensink, R. P. (2010). Variability of the glycemic response to single food products in healthy subjects. Contemporary clinical trials, 31(1), 5–11. https://doi.org/10.1016/j.cct.2009.08.001
7. Zmora, N., Suez, J., & Elinav, E. (2019). You are what you eat: Diet, health, and the gut microbiota. Nature Reviews Gastroenterology & Hepatology, 16(1), 35–56. https://doi.org/10.1038/s41575-018-0061-

SCIENTIFIC REFERENCES

2

Thank You & A Small Request

Thank you for taking the time to read this book. I truly hope it has provided you with valuable insights, practical tools, and a renewed sense of empowerment on your journey to better health.

If this book has helped you in any way, I would be so thankful if you could take one minute to leave a review. Your feedback not only helps other mothers who may be struggling with postnatal depletion, but it also allows me to continue creating resources that support women in reclaiming their vitality.

Reviews – whether a few words or a detailed reflection – make a huge difference in spreading awareness and reaching more mothers who need this information. You can leave a review on Goodreads or the website you purchased it from or simply share your thoughts with friends and family who might benefit from this book. Thank you for your support, I am eternally grateful. You along with every mother deserves to feel strong, nourished and well.

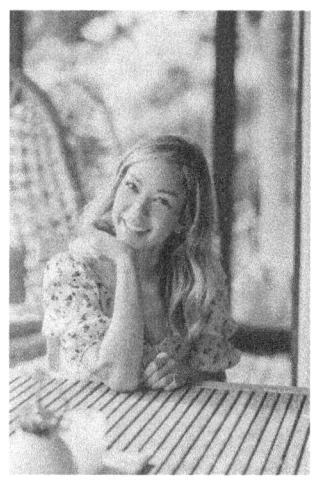

About the Author

Hi, I'm Chrissy — a university-qualified holistic nutritionist, certified health coach, nutritional medicine practitioner, gut health specialist, published writer and mum of three (including twins!). With a background in both journalism and nutrition — and an insatiable curiosity — I've spent years diving deep into the science of wellness to heal my own various health issues and help others do the same. From clients to friends and family, I've seen how powerful the right support can be and I'm passionate about making that support accessible, practical, and truly life-changing.

My health journey began out of necessity. In my 20's I became aware that my niggling health complaints were starting to snowball into an issue that I was no longer able to ignore. At my worst I was a shell of the person I was supposed to be, battling debilitating fatigue, crippling anxiety, brain fog, acne, low mood and a host of other frustrating symptoms that conventional medicine couldn't solve. After years of seeking answers from many different experts and only being offered antibiotics, anti-depressants or denials that there were any issues with my health, I continued to get sicker. It was only then, I finally realized that no one was coming to save me. It was up to me if I wanted to get better. Desperate for answers, I dove into the research, eventually uncovering the root causes and transforming my own health.

Motherhood deepened my commitment to wellness. Even though I had never felt healthier in many ways, becoming a mother revealed that some essential pieces of the puzzle were still missing — pieces that were keeping me from truly feeling my best and reaching my full potential. As a result, early motherhood felt far more stressful than it needed to be. My first postpartum experience left me feeling deeply depleted, mentally foggy, and stuck in a cycle of exhaustion where I was always tired, yet constantly wired.

Fortunately, that all changed with my twin pregnancy, I found ways to reclaim my energy and balance – and now, I feel healthier in my 40's than I did in my 20's. This is something I truly did not think was possible, and I know many others would think the same.

After many years of research, 2 university degrees, certifications in gut health, nutritional therapy and health coaching as well as helping countless people, today, I bring this same inquisitiveness and dedication to continue to share this knowledge on a much broader scale with this book.

You can connect with me on:
- https://www.sunshinehealthandnutrition.com.au
- https://www.amazon.com/stores/Chrissy-Harada/author/B0DDJ9BMKH
- https://www.instagram.com/holistic_health_nutritionist

Also by Chrissy Harada

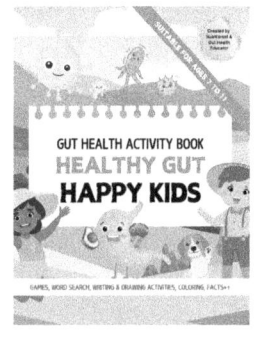

Healthy Gut, Happy Kids

Good gut health isn't just about digestion, it's the key to building a strong immune system, sharper focus, balanced mood and overall well-being. Yet gut health is often overlooked in kid's health education. This gut health activity book is here to change that, it's bursting with fun, facts, challenges & worksheets to help your little one to feel empowered to be healthier and happier.

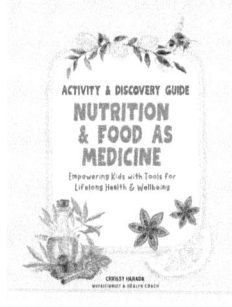

Activity & Discovery Guide: Nutrition & Food as Medicine

Make learning about nutrition fun, hands-on, and impactful! This 36-page kids' activity and discovery guide is the perfect resource for teaching children how food fuels their bodies and supports lifelong health and well-being.

www.ingramcontent.com/pod-product-compliance
Lightning Source LLC
Chambersburg PA
CBHW031144020426
42333CB00013B/508